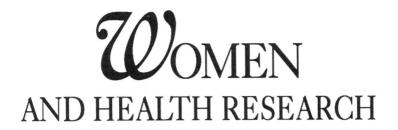

AND HEALTH RESEARCH

ETHICAL AND LEGAL ISSUES OF INCLUDING WOMEN IN CLINICAL STUDIES

VOLUME 2

Workshop and Commissioned Papers

Anna C. Mastroianni, Ruth Faden, and Daniel Federman, *Editors*

Committee on the Ethical and Legal Issues
Relating to the Inclusion of Women in Clinical Studies

Division of Health Sciences Policy

INSTITUTE OF MEDICINE

NATIONAL ACADEMY PRESS
Washington, D.C. 1994

National Academy Press • 2101 Constitution Avenue, N.W. • Washington, D.C. 20418

NOTICE: The project that is the subject of this report was approved by the Governing Board of the National Research Council, whose members are drawn from the councils of the National Academy of Sciences, the National Academy of Engineering, and the Institute of Medicine. The members of the committee responsible

This report has been reviewed by a group other than the authors according to procedures approved by a Report Review Committee consisting of members of the National Academy of Sciences, the National Academy of Engineering, and the Institute of Medicine.

The Institute of Medicine was chartered in 1970 by the National Academy of Sciences to enlist distinguished members of the appropriate professions in the examination of policy matters pertaining to the health of the public. In this, the Institute acts under both the Academy's 1863 congressional charter responsibility to be an adviser to the federal government and its own initiative in identifying issues of medical care, research, and education. Dr. Kenneth I. Shine is president of the Institute of Medicine.

This project was funded by the Office of Research on Women's Health of the National Institutes of Health (Contract No. N01-OD-2-2119) with supplemental support provided by the Ford Foundation (Grant No. 935-1335). Syntex (U.S.A.), Inc., and the Institute of Medicine also provided support for this project.

International Standard Book Number 0-309-05040-5

Volume 1 of *Women and Health Research: Ethical and Legal Issues of Including Women in Clinical Studies* and additional copies of Volume 2 are available for sale from the National Academy Press, 2101 Constitution Avenue, N.W., Box 285, Washington, D.C. 20055. Call 800-624-6242 or 202-334-3313 (in the Washington Metropolitan Area).

B313

Printed in the United States of America

The serpent has been a symbol of long life, healing, and knowledge among almost all cultures and religions since the beginning of recorded history. The image adopted as a logotype by the Institute of Medicine is based on a relief carving from ancient Greece, now held by the Staatlichemuseen in Berlin.

COMMITTEE ON THE ETHICAL AND LEGAL ISSUES RELATING TO THE INCLUSION OF WOMEN IN CLINICAL STUDIES

ANTHONY R. SCIALLI, M.D., Director, Residency Program, Georgetown University Medical Center, and Director, Reproductive Toxicology Center, Columbia Hospital for Women Medical Center, Washington, D.C.
SHELDON J. SEGAL, Ph.D., Distinguished Scientist, The Population Council, New York
WALTER J. WADLINGTON, LL.B.,* Professor of Law and of Legal Medicine, University of Virginia Law School

Study Staff

ANNA C. MASTROIANNI, Study Director
RUTH ELLEN BULGER, Division Director (until August 1993)
VALERIE P. SETLOW, Division Director (from August 1993)
ELIZABETH MEYER BOBBY, Research Associate
THELMA L. COX, Project Assistant
PHILOMINA MAMMEN, Administrative Assistant

---

* Member, Institute of Medicine

iv

Preface

In the fall of 1992, at the request of the National Institutes of Health's (NIH) Office of Research on Women's Health, the Institute of Medicine formed a committee to study the ethical and legal issues relating to the inclusion of women in clinical studies. The NIH's request was coincident with a growing perception that biomedical research had focused more on the health problems of men relative to those of women, and that women have been denied access to advances in medical diagnosis and therapy as a result of being excluded from clinical studies. With pressure from women's health advocates mounting and legislative change on the horizon, NIH requested that the committee (1) consider the ethical and legal implications of including pregnant women and women of childbearing potential in clinical studies; (2) provide practical advice for consideration by NIH, institutional review boards, and clinical investigators; and (3) examine known instances of litigation regarding injuries to research subjects and describe issues of legal liability and possible protections. Comprised of sixteen members with expertise in bioethics, law, epidemiology and biostatistics, public health policy, obstetrics and gynecology, clinical research, pharmaceutical development, social and behavioral sciences, and clinical evaluative sciences, the committee held five meetings during the one-year study. Volume 1, *Women and Health Research: Ethical and Legal Issues of Including Women in Clinical Studies,* contains the committee's final report.

The committee's report begins with an assessment of the claims regarding women's participation in clinical trials; this introduction is followed by a summary of the history of women's participation in clinical research so that readers may gain an understanding of the origins of controversy and concern surrounding this issue. An analysis of the principles of justice makes up the central chapter of the report. The committee chose to shape its report around considerations of justice in light of its understanding that calls to rectify women's alleged "underrepresentation" in clinical studies are based on concerns about the unequal distribution of the benefits of biomedical research. Subsequent chapters address the various challenges—scientific, social, ethical, and legal—to achieving justice in clinical studies. Each of the recommendations developed in these chapters flows from the central presumption embraced by the committee: that women and men should have the opportunity to participate equally in the benefits and burdens of research.

In an effort to solicit outside expertise on specific issues as well as gather input from interested individuals, the committee held an invitational workshop at the Georgetown University Conference Center on March 24–25, 1993. Speakers were invited by the committee to address such issues as recruitment and retention, liability, compensation, federal regulations, health consequences, and justice as they pertain to women's participation in clinical studies. Each speaker answered questions from the audience—a group of more than forty people from academia, industry, federal health agencies, and Congress.

This volume contains the text of the presentations given at the workshop. The presentation, *Justice and the Inclusion of Women in Clinical Studies: A Conceptual Framework*, by Professor Debra DeBruin, was expanded at the request of the committee, as this issue took on considerable importance in the committee's deliberations and final report. It is noteworthy that on the second day of the workshop, the Food and Drug Administration (FDA) announced its intention to reverse its 1977 guideline recommended the exclusion of women from early phases (Phase I and early Phase II) of drug development. Given the date of this announcement and of the formal issuance of new guidelines (July 22, 1993), the changes in FDA policy are not reflected in the presentations. Nor do the presentations take into account the June 10, 1993, passage of the NIH Revitalization Act, which also effected changes in federal policies regarding the inclusion of women in clinical studies.

Also included in this volume are additional papers commissioned by the committee. These papers address issues that were introduced at the workshop, but about which the committee felt the need for more in-depth analysis. Four of these papers focus on the research participation of women from specific racial and ethnic groups—American Indians, Alaskan Natives, Asian/Pacific Islanders, Blacks, and Latinos. In the fifth paper, the author attempts to answer the question, "Have women been 'underrepresented' in biomedical research?" through a systematic survey of clinical studies reported in the *Journal of the American Medical Association*.

The committee is indebted to the writers of this volume for their thought-provoking insights and scholarly presentation of opinions and ideas. Their work stimulated thoughtful discussion, heated debate, and sometimes even consensus. It is the committee's hope that this volume, on its own and in conjunction with Volume 1, proves to be a valuable resource to policymakers, clinical investigators, and subjects alike.

Ruth Faden, *Co-chair*
Daniel Federman, *Co-chair*

Contents

COMMISSIONED PAPERS

$\mathcal{W}$OMEN
AND HEALTH RESEARCH

Women's Participation in Clinical Research: From Protectionism to Access

Tracy Johnson and Elizabeth Fee

Nearly a decade before women's exclusion from clinical research became an issue of public scrutiny and political debate, a 1981 article documented women's underrepresentation in drug trials. The article observed that conservative Food and Drug Administration (FDA) policies which discouraged the inclusion of women of "childbearing potential" in early drug trials led to their widespread exclusion in later, Phase III testing.[1] That the article stirred so little response reflects the relative consensus at the time among researchers and federal policymakers vis a vis protectionist policies governing research on women.

In contrast, the findings of the General Accounting Office (GAO) in 1990 met with public outcry and congressional action in the form of the Women's Health Equity Act.[2] This GAO report documented that the National Institutes of Health (NIH) had made "little progress" toward implementing its 1986 policy encouraging the inclusion of women as subjects in clinical research.[3] Although NIH's records retention methods render any attempt to quantify the extent of women's exclusion difficult, press coverage has focused attention on several large-scale clinical trials with all-male study populations, e.g., the Physicians' Health Study[4] and Multiple Risk Factor Intervention Trial (aptly abbreviated as MR. FIT).[5] The mobilization of congressional women, women in the health professions, and women's advocacy organizations around this issue marks a shift in both public opinion and policy development.

CURRENT FEDERAL POLICY

Following the issuance of the 1990 GAO report, NIH promulgated a strengthened policy governing the award of federal research grants:

Applications for grants and cooperative agreements that involve human subjects are required to include minorities and both genders in study populations so that research findings can be of benefit to all persons at risk of the disease, disorder or condition under study.[6]

A 1990 NIH Policy Notice further specifies that the inclusion of women in study populations will be considered a matter of scientific and technical merit in peer review. Justifications for exclusion of either gender must be "compelling" and supported by "a strong scientific rationale."[7] As a result of these recent NIH actions, other federal agencies with jurisdiction over human research are revisiting their overlapping, and sometimes contradictory, policies.

The FDA, which oversees pharmaceutical drug testing, is presently reviewing its policies in the area.* FDA guidelines promulgated in 1977 advised that women of "childbearing potential" participate in trials only after early Phase II (efficacy and safety) trials and (female) animal reproductive studies have been completed. The guidelines provide an exception for research on life-threatening diseases.[8] For the later phase III studies, FDA lifts restrictions on women's participation and, since 1989, has advised gender (and other "subgroup") analysis of trial data.[9]

In addition, federal regulations enunciated in the Federal Policy for the Protection of Human Subjects (45 C.F.R. pt. 46) require that local institutional review boards (IRBs) ensure the ethical design of research subject to federal regulation (e.g., by the FDA) as well as research funded by the Department of Health and Human Services (DHHS). IRBs are required to assure that the "selection of subjects is equitable" and to "be particularly cognizant of the special problems of research involving vulnerable populations, such as . . . pregnant women."[10] Subpart B (which applies only to research funded by DHHS) offers "additional safeguards" for research involving fetuses, embryos, or pregnant women.[11]

Thus, at one extreme, federal (NIH) policy makes no mention of fertility

---

*On July 22, 1993, the FDA issued a new guideline titled *Guideline for the Study and Evaluation of Gender Differences in the Clinical Evaluation of Drugs.* 58 Fed. Reg. 39406–39416. The new guideline revises the section titled "Women of Childbearing Potential" in the FDA's 1977 guidelines, *General Considerations for the Clinical Evaluation of Drugs,* and describes the agency's expectations regarding inclusion of both genders as subjects of clinical trials of drugs. — Ed.

issues and dictates women's inclusion in clinical trials; at the other, federal (FDA) guidelines advise the exclusion of premenopausal women, at least during the early phases of testing. The federal regulations set forth at 45 C.F.R. pt. 46 take a middle course. They promulgate a "minimal risk" policy toward embryos/fetuses and urge explicit informed consent procedures for women, advising them of the "unforeseeable" risks of unintended pregnancy. It is small wonder that IRBs, the pharmaceutical industry, and researchers report confusion.[12] Indeed, a 1992 GAO report attributes the "underrepresentation" (ambiguously defined) of women in drug trials, as well as the lack of gender analysis, largely to imprecision in FDA guidelines.[13]

PROTECTIONIST POLICIES

Public outcry and tragedy have driven policy development in the area of research on human subjects. The original Food and Drugs Act of 1906, for example, required no safety testing prior to marketing and instead monitored drugs' strength and purity.[14] Congress passed a revised Federal Food, Drug and Cosmetic Act in 1938 only after the Elixir Sulfanilamide tragedy, which resulted in 107 poisoning deaths. The strengthened law required industry sponsors to prove drug safety before market release.[15]

Public concern and sensitivity to ethical issues in research were greatly strengthened by the Nuremberg war crime trials during the late 1940s, which revealed Nazi atrocities in human experimentation perpetrated on Jews and other "undesirables." As a result, the Nuremberg Code promulgated standards for the protection of human research subjects.[16]

During the 1960s, thalidomide-induced birth defects in Europe spurred public and congressional interest in drug development procedures in the United States. In 1962, amendments to the Food, Drug and Cosmetic Act effectively institutionalized a drug approval process resembling the one in place today. Provisions included requirements that manufacturers demonstrate safety and efficacy; that FDA collect adverse reaction reports; and that drug advertising clearly indicate associated risks as well as benefits of drug therapy.[17]

In response to new regulations as well as the threat of litigation, many pharmaceutical companies adopted increasingly conservative postures with respect to the participation of premenopausal women in clinical drug trials. Several commentators have observed that such continuing conservatism is counterintuitive given that liability incurred in the thalidomide (and subsequent) cases was due to *inadequate* drug testing and *ignored* research results which indicated the potential for reproductive harm in women.[18] Presumably, an all-male study population would not have shielded the manufacturers of thalidomide from liability claims of a drug marketed to women.

The DES and Dalkon Shield tragedies followed closely on the heels of the thalidomide disaster and coincided with the grass roots women's health movement of the 1960s and 1970s. As a result, early women's health advocates—organizations such as the Boston Women's Health Collective and the National Women's Health Network—framed the issue of women's health research as one of inappropriate *inclusion* (rather than exclusion).[19] They focused, for example, on reports that women were administered DES without their knowledge as a part of an experimental protocol.[20] Hence, these activists directed their initial efforts toward improved informed consent procedures and other protective measures for women as research participants and consumers.[21]

Public disclosure of the Tuskegee Syphilis Study during the 1970s prompted the codification of the protectionism already emergent among industry and consumer advocates. This observational study involved rural African American men with syphilis who remained in the study (untreated) well after treatment was widely available.[22] Partly in response to Tuskegee, the 1974 National Research Act called for the establishment of a National Commission for the Protection of Human Subjects of Biomedical and Behavioral Research to "identify ethical principles" and to "develop guidelines" for research involving human subjects.[23] Further impetus for creation of the National Commission was the raging political debate over abortion, artificial reproductive technologies, and fetal tissue research.[24]

In 1973, The Supreme Court case *Roe v. Wade* legalized abortion and galvanized the small but impassioned antiabortion movement in the United States.[25] Abortion politics affected not only contraceptive and abortifacient (e.g., RU486) research, but *all* research involving women of "childbearing potential." Indeed, Fletcher and Ryan have remarked on the irony that 45 C.F.R. pt. 46 grants embryos and fetuses a higher standard of protection ("minimal risk") than that accorded to children, who may in some cases participate in research involving "greater than minimal risk."[26] Others have observed that federal guidelines display more concern for (potential) fetal health than women's health.

In short, protectionist policies with respect to women's participation in clinical trials emerged from a variety of political, social, and legal forces: public outrage to unethical human experimentation, liability fears, consumer activism, and abortion politics.

ADVENT OF INCLUSIONARY POLICIES

AIDS activism concerning access to unapproved AIDS treatment therapies during the 1980s brought the first real challenge to protectionist policies.[27] The National Commission's Belmont Report (1979) had anticipated the events to come, noting that:

Beneficence thus requires that we protect against risk of harm to subjects and also that we be concerned about *the loss of substantial benefits* that might be gained from research.[28] [Emphasis added.]

In May 1987, the FDA responded to pressure from AIDS activists and issued regulations expanding access to experimental drugs used to treat "serious" and "life-threatening" illnesses.[29] Activists also lobbied loud and hard for greater public accountability with respect to awarding federal research dollars. Increased federal appropriations for AIDS research testifies to their persuasiveness.

The women's community observed the success of AIDS activists in reorienting financial and scientific resources to better address AIDS research needs. AIDS activism provided women with a language and a political strategy with which to pursue a women's health research agenda. Changing demographics provided the critical mass. Women of the baby boom generation were now of an age to be increasingly concerned about the lack of attention to their health and well-being. Dramatic increases in medical school enrollment among women during the 1970s[30] provided a vocal minority of medical professionals in the subsequent decade who questioned current priorities and policies in women health research.

Women observed that historically, medical and public health professionals have conflated women's health with reproductive and child health. Women's health needs have been subsumed under obstetrics and gynecology or addressed through maternal and child health programs. Neither the medical nor the health community perceived cardiovascular disease, for example, as "women's health," despite the fact that it is the leading cause of death for women as well as men.[31] As a result, research in nonreproductive areas seldom explored gender-linked hypotheses and often excluded women altogether.

However, pressure from female researchers within NIH resulted in a two-year U.S. Public Health Service Task Force on Women's Health Issues, which concluded in its 1985 report that:

The historical lack of research focus on women's health concerns has compromised the quality of health information available to women as well as the health care they receive.[32]

Indeed, it was the recommendations of this task force which inspired the original NIH policy to *encourage* the inclusion of women in clinical trials.

Moreover, it was women like these—from within the medical and health professions—who ultimately convinced Reps. Pat Schroeder (D-CO), Olympia Snowe (R-MA), and Henry Waxman (D-CA) to request the influential 1990 GAO report. The ensuing public outrage—particularly among women—signaled a significant shift in popular opinion. Practices and policies once presented as protective were now labeled paternalistic and discriminatory. As 1992 campaign rhetoric reminded us, these changes in perception occurred within a context of heightened gender resentment—at, for example, continued gender-based pay inequities in the work place, the erosion of abortion rights, and the Clarence Thomas-Anita Hill debacle.

Federal policies which address women's participation in clinical research were now scrutinized for bias. For instance, women's health advocates pointed to a curious section of 45 C.F.R. 46, which reads:

> When some or all of the subjects are likely to be vulnerable to coercion or undue influence, such as children, prisoners, *pregnant women*, mentally disabled persons, and economically or educationally disadvantaged persons, additional safeguards have been included in the study to protect the rights and welfare of these subjects.[33] [Emphasis added.]

One wonders what aspect of pregnancy renders women particularly vulnerable to "coercion" or "undue influence."

Women's health advocates have also observed the asymmetry in the risk/benefit analysis for research impacting male versus female reproductive potential. According to FDA guidelines, even research which has resulted in reproductive harm in male animals may go forward depending "upon the nature of the abnormalities, the dosage at which they occurred, the disease being treated, the importance of the drug, and the duration of drug administration."[34]

In contrast, a sweeping definition of "women of childbearing potential" by FDA virtually excludes all menstruating women from early testing of drug therapies. Moreover, language which implies that women "in certain institutions, e.g., prisons" might be acceptable study participants is remarkable given an ignominious history of research on institutionalized populations.[35] Critics of FDA policy have questioned whether current policy is more a reflection of gender stereotypes—female susceptibility and male invulnerability—than of good science.[36]

Since the GAO report focused on NIH policy, NIH bore the brunt of the public censure after its publication. In response to criticism, NIH officials buttressed traditional justifications for excluding women—fetal protection and liability concerns—with an argument of cost.[37] The inclusion of women in clinical research means that researchers must consider hormonal cycling and deal with larger sample sizes and recruitment "difficulties"—all of which, they argued, increase study costs.

These responses assume that the normal hormonal variations women experience throughout their menstrual cycles complicate research design by introducing an additional variable for which the researcher must control.

However, others counter that, for women, menstruation is as normal as breathing. Thus, to characterize this normal body process as "an extra variable" assumes that the male body is the norm. Critics do not dispute the existence of metabolic differences between the genders. Rather, they argue that such differences are precisely the reason that research must include both men and women.[38]

The hormonal cycling version of the cost argument fails to account for women's absence from behavioral and epidemiologic research. In these contexts, the cost argument reduces to one of sample size. Defenders of current practice argue that to represent all possible gender/racial/ethnic/age/class combinations in study populations would introduce onerous costs.[39] The counterargument holds that the goal is not to mandate the inclusion of women in each and every research activity. Instead, federal research institutions should seek to ensure that their research portfolios, when viewed in their entirety, reflect the diversity found in the U.S. population—who, after all, underwrite the studies.[40]

Certain members of the research community maintain that women are more difficult to recruit into studies.[41] While corroborating empirical evidence is often lacking, the mere perception of difficulty may itself be an obstacle. Women, they assert, require "special arrangements" such as child care and transportation. However, women's health advocates are quick to respond that women demonstrate greater health-seeking behavior than men and are generally more compliant patients and research participants.[42] On balance, perhaps the observed behavioral differences between men and women merely point to the need for gender-specific strategies to recruit and retain both genders in clinical studies, rather than pose inherent obstacles to women's inclusion.

Ultimately, the cost argument falls apart when one considers the cost of the present gaps in information about women's health. Clearly, in the absence of data on female populations, women and their health providers will continue to apply to women the research results from studies on men. This approach minimizes neither risks to women nor costs to society. Nor does it protect future children from prenatal damage.

CONCLUSION

Much as the 1970s' women's liberation movement incorporated themes of the civil rights movement, women's health advocates of the 1990s borrowed the concept of a consumer-driven research agenda from AIDS activists. Both movements have focused constructive attention on the research process. However, the challenge remains to define a policy which will minimize risks and yet allow productive research for men, women, and children. It is clear that the protectionist tradition will no longer continue unchallenged, and that women are demanding input in the evaluation of relative risks and benefits inherent in research activities. Beyond mere inclusion, women insist that their diverse health concerns should inform the formulation of the hypotheses, design, and implementation of federally funded research activities.

NOTES

1. Kinney, E. L., et al. 1981. Underrepresentation of Women in New Drug Trials: Ramifications and Remedies. *Annals of Internal Medicine.* 95(4):495–499.
2. U.S. Congress, House of Representatives. 1990. Women's Health Equity Act. H.R. 5397. 101st Congress, 2d Session.
3. U.S. General Accounting Office. 1990. National Institutes of Health: Problems in Implementing Policy on Women in Study Populations. Statement of Mark V. Nadel, Associate Director, National and Public Health Issues, Human Resources Division, before the Subcommittee on Health and the Environment, Committee on Energy and Commerce, U.S. House of Representatives. June 18. (GAO/T-HRD-90-80.)
4. Steering Committee of the Physicians Health Study Research Group. 1989. Final Report on the Aspirin Component of the On-Going Physicians Health Study. *New England Journal of Medicine.* 321:129–135.
5. Blumenthal, S. J., et al. 1991. Forging a Women's Health Research Agenda: Clinical Pharmacy Panel Report. Conference Proceedings. National Women's Health Resource Center. October. Washington, D.C.
6. National Institutes of Health (NIH) and Alcohol, Drug Abuse, and Mental Health Administration (ADAMHA). 1992. NIH/ADAMHA Inclusion of Minorities and Women as Subjects in Research: Grants and Cooperative Agreement Applications. In the application, the investigator must describe the proposed study population composition with respect to gender and minorities, include a justification of its choice, and address gender and racial/ethnic issues "in objectives of the study." Exclusion must be accompanied by a "clear, compelling rationale."
7. National Institutes of Health (NIH) and Alcohol, Drug Abuse, and Mental Health Administration (ADAMHA). 1990. NIH/ADAMHA Policy Concerning Inclusion of Women in Study Populations. NIH Guide. August 24. 19(31):18–19. (P.T. 34, II; 1014002, 1014006.)
8. U.S. Department of Health, Education and Welfare, Public Health Service, Food and Drug Administration. 1977. General Considerations for the Clinical Evaluation of Drugs. (HEW/FDA-77-3040).
9. U.S. Department of Health and Human Services, Public Health Service, Food and Drug Administration. 1989. Guideline for the Format and Content of the Clinical and Statistical Sections of New Drug Applications.
10. U.S. Department of Health and Human Services. 1991. Federal Policy for the Protection of Human Subjects. 45 C.F.R. §§ 46.101–124. Subpart A. Revised, June 18, 1991. (FR Doc. 91-14262.)
11. 45 C.F.R. §§ 46.201–211. 1991.
12. Selwitz, A. S. and Wermeling, D. P. 1992. IRB Policies and Practices: Review of Subject Population, p. 10.

13. U.S. General Accounting Office. 1992. Women's Health: FDA Needs to Ensure More Study of Gender Differences in Prescription Drug Testing. October. (GAO/HRD-93-17.)

14. Young, J. H. 1989. *Pure Food: Securing the Federal Food and Drugs Act of 1906.* Princeton, NJ: Princeton University Press.

15. Young, J. H. 1982. *The Early Years of Federal Food and Drug Control.* Madison, WI: American Institute of the History of Pharmacy.

16. National Commission for the Protection of Human Subjects of Biomedical and Behavioral Research. 1979. The Belmont Report: Ethical Principles and Guidelines for the Protection of Human Subjects of Research. April 18. (FR Doc. 79-12065.)

17. Food and Drug Administration, 1988. Evolution of U.S. Drug Law. From Test Tube to Patient: New Drug Development in the United States. Revised, March 1990. (HFI-40.)

18. Dresser, R. 1992. Wanted: Single, White Male for Medical Research. *Hastings Center Report.* January–February. 21(7):24–9.

19. The Boston Women's Health Book Collective. 1973. *Our Bodies, Ourselves.* New York: Simon & Schuster.

20. Weiss, K. 1983. Vaginal Cancer: An Iatrogenic Disease. Pp. 59–75. In *Women and Health: The Politics of Sex in Medicine.* Fee, E., ed. New York: Baywood. Pp. 59–75.

21. Faden, R., Beauchamp, T. L. and King, M. P. 1986. *A History and Theory of Informed Consent.* New York: Oxford University Press.

22. Jones, J. H. 1981. *Bad Blood: The Tuskegee Syphilis Experiment.* New York: Free Press.

23. National Research Act. July 12, 1974. (Public Law 93-348.)

24. Petchesky, R. P. 1985. *Abortion and Woman's Choice: The State, Sexuality, and Reproductive Freedom.* Boston: Northeastern University Press.

25. *Roe v. Wade,* 410 U.S. 113 (1973).

26. Fletcher, J. C. and Ryan, K. J. 1987. Federal Regulations for Fetal Research: A Case for Reform. *Law, Medicine & Health Care.* 15(3):126–138.

27. Rothman, D. J. and Edgar, H. 1992. Scientific Rigor and Medical Realities: Placebo Trials in Cancer and AIDS Research. In *AIDS: The Making of a Chronic Disease.* Fee E. and Fox D.M., eds. Berkeley: University of California Press. Pp. 194–206.

28. The Belmont Report, 1979, p. 7.

29. Rothman, D. J. and Edgar, H. 1990. New Rules for New Drugs: The Challenge of AIDS to the Regulatory Process. *Milbank Quarterly Supplement.* 68(1):111–142.

30. American Medical Association (AMA). 1991. *Women in Medicine in America: In the Mainstream.* Chicago, IL: AMA.

31. Krieger, N. and Fee, E. *Man-Made Medicine and Women's Health: The Biopolitics of Sex/Gender and Race/Ethnicity.* (In press)

32. U.S. Public Health Service. 1985. Report of the Public Health Service Task Force on Women's Health Issues. Public Health Reports. 100(1):73–106.

33. 45 C.F.R. § 46.111(a)7b (1991).

34. Food and Drug Administration. 1977, p. 11.

35. Food and Drug Administration. 1977, p. 12.
36. Kinney et al., 1981.
37. Roan, S. 1990. Sex, Ethnic Bias in Medical Research Raises Questions. *Los Angeles Times*. August 3.
38. Society for the Advancement of Women's Health Research. 1991. Annual Report: Women's Health Research—Prescription for Change. January. Washington, D.C.
39. Roan, 1990.
40. Johnson, T. 1992. Health Research that Excludes Women is Bad Science. *The Chronicle of Higher Education*. October 14. Pp. B1–2.
41. Roan, 1990.
42. Society for the Advancement of Women's Health Research, 1991.

Women in Clinical Studies: A Feminist View

Susan Sherwin

In this brief discussion, I shall appeal to certain feminist assumptions about the distribution of power and privilege in the world. Specifically, I shall simply assume agreement (and not argue for the position) that there is overwhelming evidence that women are systematically oppressed in society on the basis of their gender, and that, in many cases, gender oppression is complicated and exacerbated by other forms of oppression based on such features as race, class, ethnicity, age, religion, disabilities, or sexual orientation.[1] I also take it as well-established that the institutions responsible for the identification and delivery of health care services are implicated in the existing patterns of oppression; they play a role in the power structures of society and have, in many distinct ways, contributed to the multiple forms of oppression, and, more positively, they can play a role in dismantling oppressive systems.[2] I wish to make clear that I am not attributing malice or deliberate intent to everyone who participates in oppressive practices. I understand oppression to be systemic and endemic in society and believe that it takes conscious and persistent effort to *resist* complicity in its patterns.

I will also take it for granted that oppression is a moral and political wrong. Hence, I will be appealing to Iris Marion Young's conception of social justice, which recognizes oppression as a form of injustice. Like Young, I find most conventional standards of justice to be too narrow in their tendency to reduce justice to the question of fair distributions of identified benefits and burdens. Purely distributive approaches to justice obscure important questions of social organization and distort our understanding of the social nature of persons

11

by identifying them as atomistic, interchangeable beings. Indeed, distributive theories of justice treat as irrelevant such politically significant features of persons as their gender, race, and class. In contrast, Young's social justice conception recognizes the importance of attending to these kinds of considerations in order to correct the effects of oppressive practices that arise from the biases inherent in sexism, racism, classism, and so on. Treating people as if they are equally situated with respect to power and privilege when they are not is a way of maintaining existing power structures. Understanding justice as social justice, defined as including concern for matters of domination and oppression, invites us to respond to the crippling biases and differing access to power that underlie systematic patterns of oppression. Even when our focus is purely distributive, it is important to raise questions about the social context in which distributions are carried out.

Thus, when we are trying to decide on a matter of social policy with respect to an oppressed group, this conception of social justice requires us to investigate how the proposed practice is likely to affect current patterns of domination and oppression in society: i.e., is it likely to worsen or improve the existing levels of oppression in society?[3] Among other ethical questions, we need to ask of each practice or policy reviewed, whose interests does it serve and whose does it harm? In the current context, where the task is to decide about policy regarding the inclusion of women in clinical studies, the ethical questions raised should include questions about how the proposed policy will affect the oppressed status of all women and, more specifically, how it will affect the status of women who are multiply oppressed by virtue of the intersection of gender with their race, class, age, and so on. By this measure, we can identify several specific areas of feminist concern, including: (1) some or all women may be unjustly excluded from some studies and suffer as a result; (2) women may be unjustly enrolled in studies that expose them to risk without offering appropriate benefits; (3) the research agenda may be unresponsive to the interests of oppressed groups; and (4) most generally, the process by which research decisions are made and carried out may maintain and promote oppressive practices. I will expand on each of these concerns in turn.

(1) The exclusion of women from important clinical studies is the best known of the problems of injustice identified as falling within the scope of the topic of women's role in clinical studies. Historically, many studies of diseases that are common to both sexes have systematically excluded women from participation, so the necessary data for guiding treatment decisions for women are unavailable.[4] Women's health care must often be based on untested inferences from data collected about men, but because there are important physiological differences between women and men, such inferences cannot always be presumed to be reliable; and, even when some data are collected about women's responses to the treatment in question, we may lack information about how a proposed treatment will affect specific groups of women (e.g., those who

are disabled, elderly, or poor). Even according to traditional distributive conceptions of justice, it is clear that this sort of discrimination is unjust and bound to result in less effective health care for (some) women than for comparable men because the knowledge base which guides health care practices is unfairly skewed; if we accept the view that well-designed clinical studies are beneficial for a population, then the systematic exclusion of women from such studies must be seen as disadvantaging them unfairly. A social justice approach that is sensitive to matters of oppression helps us to recognize that this disadvantage is not random or accidental, but is a result and further dimension of women's generally oppressed status in society. According to the distributive models of justice, women ought to be represented proportionately to their health risk in any clinical studies likely to be of benefit to subject populations. The social justice model I am proposing allows us to argue the stronger claim that in order to counteract the disadvantage from which they begin, those who are currently oppressed in society should have a privileged place in studies that are likely to be of specific benefit to members of the group investigated.

(2) It is important, however, not to translate this call for greater research attention toward women and other oppressed groups into a wholesale endorsement of the use of members of oppressed groups as research subjects in all studies without qualification. Clinical trials often expose subjects to significant risk, discomfort, or inconvenience without offering any special benefits to either the subjects or the groups from which they are recruited; in many trials, other, more privileged subjects would have served equally well except for the fact that the well-being of such people is more highly valued by society. Many shameful events in the history of clinical research testify to the ease with which researchers exploit the vulnerability of oppressed or devalued members of society for the ultimate benefit of others; far from demonstrating an interest in providing effective care for the group in question, in these cases the choice of subjects reflects the perceived expendability of members of the subject group.[5] Various approaches have been pursued to guard against the exploitative abuse of research subjects. Ethical guidelines recommend getting informed, voluntary consent from subjects and taking special precautions with groups that are recognized as being especially vulnerable to exploitation, such as children, people who are very ill or infirm, prisoners, those with severe mental handicaps, and those who are living in institutions. The guidelines usually restrict the use of subjects from groups recognized as being most readily exploited to studies that are of explicit benefit to that group. These restrictions should be extended to encompass oppressed groups: they also constitute a group that is at particular risk of exploitation, since society values them less than other groups and so is more inclined to expose them to risk. It is important to ensure that oppressed people are not included in research studies merely on the basis of the unjust belief that risks or inconvenience are less significant when they occur to devalued individuals. Clinical studies which propose to recruit women or members of other

oppressed groups should be required to demonstrate that the results produced will be of specific benefit to the individuals or to the group in question.[6]

(3) Feminists raise several ethical questions about the content of research agendas and the process for setting them:

(3a) Although the research agenda regarding women's health needs has historically neglected many important questions, there has been a substantial body of research directed at gaining control over women's reproduction. In fact, this is the one area of study where women have received a disproportionately large share of research attention. For example, almost all contraceptive research has explored means of controlling women's fertility.[7] Similarly, efforts to relieve infertility have focused on procedures that can be done to women—even when the infertility is associated with such male conditions as low sperm count.[8] As a result, a disproportionate share of the burden, risks, expenses, and responsibility for managing fertility now belongs to women, because that is where the knowledge base is. Again, this imbalance in available knowledge can be recognized as unjust by traditional distributive justice measures, but a richer social justice perspective provides further indications of injustice in light of the fact that women's oppressed status is inseparable from their traditionally assigned roles in the spheres of sexuality and reproduction. The concentration of medical attention on women's reproductive role not only assumes the conventional view that women are, by nature, to be responsible and available for reproductive activities; it also legitimizes, reinforces, and further entrenches such views and the attitudes that accompany them. Moreover, the knowledge obtained through these studies is sometimes used by those with more power in society to regulate and control women's fertility, e.g., through population control programs and those that sterilize women who are deemed to be unsuitable mothers.[9] Clearly, not all women are affected equally by the knowledge produced by studies into women's reproduction. Women who are multiply oppressed, i.e., those who are poor, belong to racial minorities, suffer from mental illness, or live in a Third World country, are at far higher risk of imposed contraception or sterilization than are privileged white women; at the same time, new reproductive technologies aimed at facilitating conception are usually made available only to the most affluent and advantaged women in society.

(3b) Studies into the control of women's reproduction also raise another area of feminist concern, namely, the absence of clear guidelines to distinguish between therapy, innovative practice, and research. Historically and currently many women have paid very high prices when unsafe treatments are provided as means of obtaining control over some aspect of their reproductive lives. From contraceptives (Dalkon Shield, early doses of birth control pills), through drugs prescribed in pregnancy (DES, thalidomide), to the ever-expanding practices in the area of new reproductive technologies, treatments have been developed and offered to women as therapy without adequate prior clinical studies to establish their safety and effectiveness. Clinical studies are governed by regulations ensuring patients receive detailed information and careful monitoring; further protection is provided by the demands for peer review before the initiation of a study. No such control exists in untested therapies that may be offered as innovative treatment, or, sometimes, as conventional treatment. Because oppression involves a society's devaluing of the interests of those who are oppressed, there is significant danger that victims of oppression may face higher risks of harm when they are singled out for new, unproven treatments. When dealing with treatments offered solely to members of an oppressed group, it is especially important, then, to ensure that patients' interests are protected. Regulations demanding testing and monitoring before therapies are mass marketed to some specific oppressed group may be necessary to improve safety standards.

(3c) A justice model that concerns itself with oppression also provides grounds for objecting to the fact that almost the entire health research budget is absorbed by clinical studies directed at conditions that threaten those who are most privileged in society. Moreover, the bulk of the health research agenda is defined around a model of crisis intervention, rather than prevention. Thus, even though the links between poverty and illness are well known, efforts are concentrated in developing ways of responding to illness rather than avoiding it in the first place. Other specific health concerns of those who are most marginalized in society tend to be virtually ignored: e.g., there is little research into lupus, a disease found three times as often in black women as in the general population;[10] and despite the flurry of research attention provoked by AIDS, the investigation of AIDS in women has also been neglected, perhaps because it is believed that few white women are at risk of contracting AIDS, though African American women face a risk 12 times higher.[11] In addition, too many clinical studies explore expensive, highly technological solutions which, even if successful, will be accessible to only a small proportion of the population within developed countries—they are virtually useless in a global perspective of health needs. In general, research agendas reflect the interests, power, and privilege of the elites who set them; they are seldom defined by the health needs or interests of those who are most marginalized in society. It is no surprise, then, that clinical studies tend to produce knowledge that strengthens the health and opportunity of those who are already well placed in society while ignoring the needs of the disadvantaged, leaving them in ever weaker relative positions. If we want to recognize and respond to existing patterns of oppression we must go beyond the questions of who to include or exclude in research studies and investigate which studies are conducted and which are not pursued.

(4) Therefore, if we are serious about eradicating oppression, we must begin by challenging the process by which research agendas are set and research programs are carried out. Some feminists have argued that we need to rethink current views of research as an objective, technical activity in which investigators belong to an elite group of knowledgeable scientists and subjects are regarded

as their passive research tools; they propose alternate conceptions of research as a collegial activity in which subjects and investigators negotiate the terms of participation to achieve a shared commitment to the success of the activity.[12] Research is not separate from other practices of society, and it is certainly not automatically immune from the poisonous effects of bias. If clinical research is to respond fully to the demands of justice, investigators will need to develop ways to be more inclusive and less elitist in all stages of their studies. They might, for example, adapt models of participatory democracy, in which those who have a stake in the research help to formulate priorities. In order to begin to counteract the disadvantage that oppression creates for its victims, members of oppressed groups should, whenever possible, be included, not only as subjects, but also as investigators and active participants in the deliberations.

NOTES

1. I shall not provide any evidence for this belief since the literature is filled with detailed analysis of the systematic ways in which women are disadvantaged economically, socially, legally, politically, physically, and culturally. The account of oppression underlying my interpretation of the empirical data about women's disadvantaged status and choices as constituting oppression has been provided by Iris Marion Young, *Justice and the Politics of Difference* (Princeton: Princeton University Press, 1990). Young identifies five conditions as characterizing oppression, whether they appear singly or in combination: exploitation, marginalization, powerlessness, cultural imperialism, and violence.

2. See, for example, Barbara Ehrenreich and Deirdre English, *For Her Own Good: 150 Years of the Experts' Advice to Women* (Garden City, N.Y.: Anchor Books, 1979); Elizabeth Fee, ed., *Women and Health: The Politics of Sex in Medicine* (Farmindgale, N.Y.: Bayood, 1983); Sue Fisher, *In the Patient's Best Interest: Women and the Politics of Medical Decisions* (New Brunswick, N.J.: Rutgers University Press, 1986); Cesar A. Periles and Lauren S. Young, eds., *Too Little, Too Late: Dealing with the Health Needs of Women in Poverty* (New York: Harrington Park Press, 1988); Alexandra Dundas Todd, *Intimate Adversaries: Cultural Conflict Between Doctors and Women Patients* (Philadelphia: University of Pennsylvania Press, 1989); Evelyn C. White, ed., *The Black Women's Health Book: Speaking for Ourselves* (Seattle: Seal Press, 1990).

3. This argument is spelled out in greater detail in Susan Sherwin, *No Longer Patient: Feminist Ethics and Health Care* (Philadelphia: Temple University Press, 1992).

4. Several examples of such exclusions are provided by Rebecca Dresser, "Wanted: Single, White Male for Medical Research," *Hastings Center Report* 22(1):24–29, 1992.

5. Nazi studies on concentration camp prisoners and the Tuskegee Syphilis Study are two of the most notorious examples in this category.

6. See Sherwin, *No Longer Patient*, pp. 159–165.

7. Gena Corea, *The Hidden Malpractice: How American Medicine Mistreats Women*, updated edition (New York: Harper Colophon Books, 1985), pp. 130–188.

8. Renate D. Klein, *Infertility: Women Speak Out About Their Experiences of Reproductive Medicine* (London: Pandora Press, 1989).

9. Kathleen McDonnell, ed., *Adverse Effects: Women and the Pharmaceutical Industry* (Toronto: The Women's Press, 1986).

10. Vida Labrie Jones, "Lupus and Black Women: Managing a Complex Chronic Disability," in White, ed., *The Black Women's Health Book.*

11. In Angela Y. Davis, "Sick and Tired of Being Sick and Tired: The Politics of Black Women's Health," in White, ed., *The Black Woman's Health Book.*

12. See, for example, Sandra Harding, *Whose Science? Whose Knowledge?* (Ithaca: Cornell University Press, 1991).

Ethical Issues Related to the Inclusion of Pregnant Women in Clinical Trials (I)

John Robertson

Researchers, institutional review boards (IRBs) and others reviewing clinical research including pregnant women must assess the effect of proposed research on the pregnant woman, on the developing fetus, and on the child whom the fetus, if carried to term, will become. In most instances concern with fetal effects is not by virtue of the fetus's interests in its own right, but by virtue of the effect which prenatal interventions affecting the fetus will have on offspring.

A set of guidelines for such research was developed by the National Commission for the Protection of Human Subjects of Biomedical and Behavorial Science Research in 1974. These guidelines were incorporated into federal regulations for research with human subjects in 1975, and continue to apply today (45 C.F.R. §§ 46.201–46.211). They are generally sound with the specifications and modifications discussed below.

THE PREGNANT WOMAN AS SUBJECT

Both the National Commission and the federal regulations distinguish clinical research involving pregnant women on the basis of whether the woman or the fetus is the subject of the research. In each case they make a further distinction between research that is therapeutic—the purpose of the activity is to meet the "health needs of the mother" or "the health needs of the particular fetus"—and research that is nontherapeutic.[1] The amount of risk which may be

18

accepted depends on this set of distinctions.

Therapeutic: To Meet the Health Needs of the Mother

Pregnant women may participate in clinical research where the "purpose of the activity is to meet the health needs of the mother" regardless of the degree of risk to the fetus and offspring. If the purpose of the research is not to meet her health needs, she may participate only if "the risk to the fetus is minimal." While this rule is generally sound, it conceals some problems. The main problem concerns the broad phrase "health needs of the mother." Consider an established treatment for a disease or condition that is safe and effective for women whenever it is given, but also has a very high risk of affecting future offspring if given during pregnancy. Ethical judgment of whether the woman should be able to have the treatment during pregnancy will depend not merely on whether the treatment will affect her "health," but also on the burdens and benefits to her of having treatment during pregnancy or after. The type of benefit to her alone is not determinative, but the magnitude is. The more minor the benefits the less discretion the woman should have to accept treatment, if there is any risk beyond minimal to offspring.

Such a standard requires weighing the importance to the woman of the health need in question versus the risk to offspring. Treating morning sickness or a cold during pregnancy is certainly a health need. But if the drug used to treat those conditions is teratogenic, it would be unethical to take it even though it is directed at treating her "health." If this is true about established therapies, then it is even more true about experimental therapies. If use of an experimental drug poses more than minimal risks to the fetus and offspring, a woman should have even less of a moral right to take such a drug to treat a cold, morning sickness, or any condition that is not life-threatening or very serious, where the primary purpose of the research is to meet her health needs. Thus a researcher, an IRB, or other review body should make a judgment about the degree of the benefits or burdens of taking or forgoing the experimental treatment relative to the harm to the fetus and offspring if it is given. A purpose of treating the "health needs" alone of the pregnant woman is not ethical when the benefits to her are greatly outweighed by the risks to fetus and offspring. The current federal regulations are overbroad to the extent that they would permit such research to occur.

Nontherapeutic Research: Not Meeting the Health Needs
of the Pregnant Woman

Where the purpose of clinical research involving a pregnant woman is not to meet her health needs, the regulations limit such research only to instances where "the risk to the fetus is minimal." The implicit ethical assessment is that a pregnant woman may not harm expected offspring when there is no health benefit to her.

The first thing to note about this regulation is the ambiguity inherent in "risk to the fetus." Strictly speaking, "risk to the fetus" could be interpreted to mean only those risks that will prevent the fetus from being born alive, i.e., that might induce miscarriage. But that meaning does not make sense because women do not have moral duties to bring previable fetuses to term. Hence, they would be morally entitled to engage in activity which has a risk of inducing miscarriage, because the fetus itself lacks interests or rights. Except for persons who view the fetus as a person or moral subject in its own right, the moral concern with research or other impacts on fetuses arises because fetuses generally go to term and become offspring. More than minimal risk to a fetus is of ethical concern because of the impact which that risk will have on the resulting child. Thus it is necessary to understand "risk to the fetus" as "risk to the fetus that will be carried to term." The only qualification to this understanding would arise with research involving viable fetuses. In those cases risk to the fetus might also be of concern because it prevented an entity with interests in itself from being born.[2]

Thus understood, the point of the regulation is to protect expected offspring from experimental prenatal harms that are not justified by important health needs of the woman. The woman is not free to sacrifice the interests of expected offspring by her interest in serving the needs of science or of other women. She is free to make a martyr of herself, but she is not free to make a martyr of her children, whether the martydom occurs by prenatal or postnatal conduct.

This understanding of the regulation is ethically sound. The only argument against it would be the claim made by some feminists that a pregnant woman should be free to do what she wants with her body, and that any restrictions on her behavior is an intolerable restriction of her freedom. The very issue being discussed shows that this position is unsound, even if one believes that coercive state interventions to prevent prenatal harm to offspring are rarely justified on policy grounds. The regulation, however, is ethically sound. No one, not even the pregnant woman, has a moral right to engage in experimental clinical research not necessary to meet her own substantial health needs when there will be a major impact on offspring.

THE FETUS AS SUBJECT

Clinical research involving pregnant women may also be directed at the fetus as the subject of the research. Again, the major ethical distinction in this category is between therapeutic and nontherapeutic fetal research, the former being cases where the "purpose of the activity [is] to meet the health needs of the particular fetus" (45 C.F.R. § 46.208(a)).

Therapeutic: To Meet the Health Needs of the Fetus

The federal regulations permit research with the fetus as subject when "the purpose of the activity is to meet the health needs of the particular fetus and the fetus will be placed at risk only to the minimum extent necessary to meet such needs."

This standard is ethically unexceptional once the ambiguity mentioned earlier in "health needs of the fetus" is resolved. The term in this context would apply to procedures that will enable the fetus to survive, i.e., come to term, and survive in a healthy or undamaged way. Thus experimental procedures designed to prevent or treat handicap or disease in offspring would be permitted, because the health needs of the fetus include the health needs of the child that the fetus will become. Prenatal procedures on the fetus are necessary to safeguard the welfare of offspring. Thus experimental *in utero* fetal surgery to correct diaphragmatic hernia in the fetus may be done because of the impact which that condition will have on offspring.

Note that there is no obligation to include the fetus in experimental research. Parents have no duty to subject their fetuses and offspring to experimental procedures, even when there is no alternative treatment available, precisely because it is experimental and thus not clearly a benefit. On the other hand, parents should be free to have experimental *in utero* therapies used when they reasonably believe that the benefits of the procedure to offspring outweigh the risks.

Nontherapeutic Fetal Research: Not to Meet the Fetus's Health Needs

The federal regulations restrict research not directed to meet the health needs of the fetus to situations in which "the risk to the fetus imposed by the research is minimal and the purpose of the activity is the development of important biomedical knowledge which cannot be obtained by other means" (45 C.F.R. § 46.209(b)).

This rule is ethically sound—indeed, is morally obligatory—in situations in which the pregnancy may or will go to term. In that case research not designed to benefit offspring would occur that has more than minimal risk of harming offspring. Because parents have no right to harm their offspring, whether by prenatal or postnatal conduct, they have no more right to include their offspring in prenatal experiments that carry a risk of harm than they do to include them in postnatal research. Note, however, that they would have the right to include them in minimally risky research on the ground that no ethical or legal duty would be violated in doing so. However, this regulation is not justified in situations where the pregnancy will not go to term. In such cases, strictly speaking, there is no risk of harm to the fetus, because a previable fetus is insufficiently developed to have interests in its own right, and thus cannot be harmed. The National Commission, however, took the position that all fetuses should be treated equally—those going to be aborted should be treated the same as those going to term. Under the Commission's understanding no research could be done on fetuses going to be aborted that could not be done on fetuses going to term. Treating all fetuses the same overlooks the fact that nontherapeutic research on fetuses going to term could affect the interests of offspring, whereas research on fetuses to be aborted cannot hurt future offspring, much less previable fetuses, which are nonsentient and do not have interests.

There is one possible risk with nontherapeutic research on fetuses going to be aborted that is of ethical concern. That risk is that the woman who consents to that research might change her mind about abortion after the experimental procedure has begun. If so, research begun with no intention of harming offspring could end up harming children who are later born. Of course, once the experimental procedure has begun, the woman might be reluctant to change her mind precisely because of risk of harm to offspring. To make research ethically acceptable on fetuses going to be aborted, the experimental procedure should be administered shortly before the abortion or in other circumstances in which it is very clear that the pregnancy will in fact be terminated, and that the woman has had sufficient opportunity to contemplate that decision. Researchers and reviewers should assure that this condition is met.

NOTES

1. § 46.207(a); § 46.208(a).
2. This statement assumes a certain view of why viable fetuses are protected. If protection is based on sentience alone—an interest in avoiding pain and suffering—they may not also have an interest in coming to term.

Ethical Issues Related to the Inclusion of Pregnant Women in Clinical Trials (II)

Bonnie Steinbock

More than a billion drug prescriptions are written every year, there is unlimited self-administration of "over-the-counter" drugs, and approximately 500 new pharmaceutical products are introduced annually (Briggs et al., 1983, cited in Elias & Annas, 1987, p. 196). Moreover, a surprisingly high number of pregnant women use legal drugs; 40 percent in the first trimester, according to one study (Heinonen et al., 1977, cited in Elias and Annas, 1987, p. 196). These facts lead to the conclusion that "the potential for drug teratogenicity is thus truly remarkable" (Elias and Annas, 1987, p. 196).

Much information about the pharmacology of the maternal–fetal unit has been derived from animal studies, but it is extremely difficult to predict whether observations made in animals will have relevance to human beings. For example, preliminary testing of the rubella vaccine in monkeys indicated that the vaccine did not cross the placenta. However, when human studies were undertaken with women about to undergo abortions, it was found that the vaccine virus did cross the placenta and infect the fetus. Thalidomide is another dramatic example that negative animal data do not prove that a drug is innocuous to humans. This presents a dilemma. If we include pregnant women in clinical trials, we risk exposing fetuses to the risk of teratogenicity. If we exclude pregnant women from clinical trials, we will not have information about the effects of various drugs on the maternal/placental/fetal unit. We must therefore steer between Scylla and Charybdis, and we need appropriate guidelines to help.

This issue was addressed by the National Commission for the Protection of

Human Subjects of Biomedical and Behavioral Research, the first of whose mandates was to review and report on research involving living fetuses. The result was a report, *Research on the Fetus.* Among its recommendations were the following: nontherapeutic research on the pregnant woman or on the fetus *in utero* may be conducted or supported, provided it will impose minimal or no risk to the fetus, the woman's informed consent has been obtained, and the father has not objected (*Research on the Fetus,* pp. 73–76).

Several key concepts are included in this recommendation. The first is nontherapeutic research, that is, research that does not benefit the research subject, in this case, either the pregnant woman or the fetus. Placing restrictions on the use of pregnant women in nontherapeutic research limits their freedom of choice, but it cannot be said to harm them as individuals. Women taken as a class may be harmed by the exclusion of women from clinical trials. Indeed, such exclusion is likely to affect adversely society as a whole, as important knowledge that might have been acquired may not be gained. The situation is quite different for therapeutic research, to which I will return shortly.

The next key concept is that of risk to the fetus. The National Commission required that the risk to the fetus from the research be minimal or nonexistent. It maintained that all fetuses should be protected from potentially harmful research, regardless of whether they were going to be aborted or going to be born: ". . . the same principles apply whether or not abortion is contemplated; in both cases, only minimal risk is acceptable" (*Research on the Fetus,* p. 66). This requirement was referred to as "the principle of equality."

I disagree. In my view, because of the difference between children and early-gestation fetuses, it is crucially important whether the woman is going to abort or going to term. Early-gestation fetuses are not sentient or conscious or aware of anything. No matter what is done to them, they feel nothing. Nonsentient fetuses cannot be harmed in the way that sentient beings can be harmed; that is, they can't be hurt or made to suffer. Treatment that would cause a sentient being to experience pain is not necessarily harmful to nonsentient fetuses.

However, pain isn't the only way in which a being can be harmed. What if a fetus is exposed to substances that prevent it from developing normally, such as the rubella virus, thalidomide, alcohol, and so forth. Here, however, the harm is not to the fetus, but to the born child. It is the child who must go through life deaf and mentally retarded when the fetus has been harmed by prenatal exposure to rubella. It is the child who must go through life without limbs when the fetus has been harmed by thalidomide. It is the child who must go through life with learning disabilities when the fetus has been harmed by prenatal exposure to alcohol. If the woman aborts in the first trimester, before the fetus becomes sentient or conscious, there is no one who can be harmed. That is why a woman who plans to abort has only her own health to consider regarding drinking or smoking, while the woman who plans to go to term has the health of her future child to consider, as well as her own health.

If this is right, then it makes no sense to insist, as did most of the Commissioners, that no procedures should be applied to a fetus-to-be-aborted that would not be applied to a fetus-going-to-term. The reason for banning potentially harmful nontherapeutic research on fetuses-going-to-term is not to protect the fetus per se, but rather to protect the future child. If the woman is going to abort, there won't be any future child, and literally no one who can be harmed or protected. Moreover, if women who are scheduled to abort are willing to participate in clinical trials, and give their informed consent, much useful information that will serve to protect future children may be gained. What if the woman is going to term? In this case, the interests of the surviving child must be considered. Could there be any objection if there are only minimal or no risks to the future child? Paul Ramsey opposed *all* nontherapeutic research on children, on the ground that they have not given informed consent (Ramsey, 1976). Richard McCormick thinks that some nontherapeutic research on children can be justified, and that parents can give proxy consent for their children where there is no discernible risk or undue comfort. Proxy consent is morally legitimate insofar as it represents what the child *ought* to choose—and everyone ought to be willing to participate in experiments that benefit the human community (McCormick, 1974). Both Ramsey and McCormick regard informed consent, either given directly or through a proxy, as morally required. However, it is hard to see the point of requiring informed consent in situations when it is literally impossible. Surely the important point is whether the research is likely to harm the children, either after or before birth. I am assuming that the question of whether research will impose more than minimal risks upon offspring is an objective and scientific matter. If so, then this is not a matter for potential participants in nontherapeutic research to assess. Rather, it is the duty of researchers to determine if the research poses more than minimal risks to offspring. If it does not, then there doesn't seem to be any objection to it.

What if the risks are either significant or unknown? Should a woman be allowed to expose her not-yet-born child to such risks? It is difficult to imagine a situation in which a woman would want to expose her future child to risks, when there is no benefit either to herself or to the child. But imagine a woman with a Mother Theresa complex. She wants to volunteer for medical research to help humanity, and she's willing to take the risk that it might harm either her or her baby. It seems entirely reasonable for us to tell her that while she is permitted to take such risks on her own behalf, she is not entitled to impose such risks on her not-yet-born child. After all, preventing her from participating in an experiment isn't infringing her bodily integrity. It isn't monitoring her lifestyle. So I see no objection to regulations preventing pregnant women who plan to go to term from participating in risky nontherapeutic research.

Restrictions are harder to justify where the research offers a potential benefit to the pregnant woman. Experimental therapy may offer the only hope to individuals who are sick and cannot be helped by tested methods, such as people who have AIDS. They have a direct personal interest in being included in clinical trials. Not allowing them to participate does not merely infringe their autonomy and right to decide for themselves; it may foreclose the only hope they have of survival. It seems, therefore, that it would be wrong to exclude pregnant women who are not going to term from experimental trials that might benefit them.

What about women who wish to continue their pregnancies? I don't think it matters much if the therapy is experimental or conventional. The question is the same: does a woman who is planning on going to term have the right to undergo therapy that poses a risk to her fetus?

A recent story in the *New York Times* described an Italian woman who refused cancer therapy out of concern that it would harm the fetus she was carrying. She was willing to die in order to avoid harming her fetus. If one views the fetus as having the same status as a born child, then this may seem like a noble act of self-sacrifice. (This is how the Vatican regards it. I believe that they are taking steps to canonize her.) My own view is that her refusal of therapy is certainly permissible, but not morally required. No one is morally required to sacrifice her own life or health to sustain the life of a fetus (Thomson, 1971).

But what if the therapy isn't likely to be lethal to the fetus, but rather risks causing it to be born with severe handicaps? If the risk is great enough, and the handicaps severe enough, terminating the pregnancy might be morally required. For abortion is not a harm to the nonconscious fetus, but being born with very severe impairments may be unfair to the child (Steinbock and McClamrock, in press).

What if the potential benefit is to the fetus, that is, the surviving child? In general, parents have the responsibility for deciding whether to impose experimental treatment on their minor children. Similarly, the prospective parents should be allowed to decide, within comparable limits, whether the potential benefits to the fetus outweigh the risks. However, there is one glaring difference between the two situations. Prenatal treatment of a fetus can be done only through the body of its mother. So the risks to her are an important part of the decision. In recent years, fetal therapy and surgery has grown by leaps and bounds. In one dramatic case (which by now has no doubt been repeated several times) a surgeon removed a pre-viable fetus from the uterus, repaired his diaphragmatic hernia, put the fetus back in the womb, and delivered him six weeks later by cesarean section (Kolata, 1990). The mother had no obligation to try the therapy, given the risks and burdens to her from two cesareans and six weeks of enforced bed rest, especially since it was very experimental and carried no guarantee of success. Even if such therapy should become "routine," it still should never be compulsory. But neither should anyone deny a pregnant woman the chance to save her baby's life.

Finally, I'd like to consider the role of the woman's partner in making these decisions. By partner, I mean the man who is not only the genetic father, but who also intends to be a rearing parent. It seems to me that if the woman is planning to abort, the man should have no say in whether she participates in a clinical trial. For while a man has a legitimate interest in the well-being of his offspring, if the woman decides to abort, there won't be any offspring. The decision to participate in a clinical trial belongs solely to the pregnant woman.

A man would have a legitimate interest in preventing a woman who did not plan to abort from participating in nontherapeutic research that posed some risk to the not-yet-born child. However, there's a strong case for society's banning pregnant women who plan to go to term from such clinical trials, whether or not the father objects.

Men have legitimate interests in the health of their not-yet-born children. It is not unreasonable for them to be concerned if their pregnant wives smoke or abuse alcohol or drugs. It seems unfair that a man who intends to parent a child should have to stand by and watch behavior that risks harming his future child. He is certainly justified in trying to persuade his wife to get treatment, for the sake of their baby. He might even be justified in coercing her to get treatment, since this will benefit both her and the baby. But he would not be justified in preventing his pregnant wife from getting therapy necessary for her own life and health, to protect the future child. Being a Good—or Splendid—Samaritan may be noble and praiseworthy; it is not something one individual has any right to demand of another.

REFERENCES

Briggs, G. G., Bodendorter T. W., Freeman R. K., et al. 1983. Drugs in Pregnancy and Lactation: A Reference Guide to Fetal and Neonatal Risk. Baltimore: Williams & Wilkins.

Elias, S., and Annas, G. 1987. Reproductive Genetics and the Law. Chicago: Year Book Medical Publishers.

Heinonen, O. P., Slone, D., and Shapiro, S. 1977. Birth Defects and Drugs in Pregnancy. Littleton, Mass.: Publishing Science Group.

Kolata, G. 1990. Lifesaving surgery on a fetus works for the first time. *The New York Times,* Thursday, May 31, A1.

McCormick, R. A. 1974. Proxy consent in the experimentation situation. *Perspectives in Biology and Medicine* 18:2–20.

The National Commission for the Protection of Human Subjects of Biomedical and Behavioral Research. 1975. Research on the Fetus: Report and Recommendations (cited as Research on the Fetus), DHEW Pub. No. (OS) 76–127.

Ramsey, P. 1976. The enforcement of morals: Nontherapeutic research on children. *Hastings Center Report* 6(4):21–30.
Steinbock, B., and McClamrock, R. In press. When is birth unfair to the child? *Bioethics*.
Thomson, J. J. 1971. A defense of abortion. *Philosophy and Public Affairs* 1:1.

Ethical Issues Related to the Inclusion of Women of Childbearing Age in Clinical Trials

Jonathan D. Moreno

In this brief paper I will discuss the ethical issues associated with the enrollment of women of reproductive potential in clinical trials. I should say at the outset that I believe that women in the referenced population should not be excluded as a class from participation in clinical trials or studies. In the policy I recommend, the exclusion of individual members would have to satisfy the burden of argument that risks are intolerable. In other words, I favor reversing the traditional presumption from exclusion to inclusion.

Without prejudicing the question of recruiting pregnant women as subjects, it should be appreciated that the historic basis for our largely exclusionary policy has been concern about fetal protection.[1] The extension of protectionism from pregnant women to all women of reproductive potential was, I believe, the result of intellectual lassitude, defensive legalism, and a misplaced sense of obligation.[2] While it might be argued that the prospect of increased research costs has also been a factor, I do not believe that such estimates were attempted until quite recently, when the prospect of a policy change became serious.

There are a number of considerations that support the reform of current policy toward a presumption of inclusion of women of reproductive potential as research subjects. These considerations can be related to three ethical principles that have been viewed as the appropriate analytic framework for questions concerning the morality of clinical trials: respect for persons, beneficence, and justice.[3]

The most powerful (if not persuasive) argument one could make against exposing women and their possible offspring to the risks of research participation is that we should not expose anyone to unnecessary risk in the name of science.

But in our society we have in effect concluded that research involving human subjects should go forward when participation is voluntary, the risk appears to be minimal, and the foreseeable benefits to others, if not in all cases the subject, are substantial.[4]

What seems to have distinguished policies concerning research involving women of reproductive potential from research involving other kinds of subjects is the prospect of harm to possible children. Legal issues aside, I can think of three moral grounds for such policies: that possible children cannot consent, that the interests of later generations should be protected by earlier ones, and that biologically mediated risks to future human beings are uniquely unacceptable.

The primary purpose of consent policies has been the protection of research subjects. The prospective subject in the studies in question is the woman, not the possible child. In the case of research involving young children, parents have been regarded as the most appropriate sources of permission for research participation. There is also a special class of *potential* children or fetuses (as against *possible* children, who are those prior to conception or individuation or "brain birth" or viability), who could be affected by a woman's participation in research. Consonant with policies concerning children as subjects, when research involving pregnant women has been permitted, potential parents have been regarded as the appropriate decision makers concerning the acceptability of fetal risk, except when a risk–benefit analysis applied to the woman fetus pair is patently unfavorable.

Future generations will include women as well as children. Thus the interests of future generations include improved treatment of diseases affecting women. Even if there was reason to think that clinical trials create a serious conflict between the interests of future women and future children (interests which must surely be seen as complementary), the interests of the former could not *a priori* be dismissed in favor of those of the latter.

Finally, one might claim that there is something "worse" about biologically mediated risks as compared to other risks that social action creates for future generations. I do not know what sense to give such a claim, and I do not think that it can be defended without mystifying biological, as against social, relations.

I will now turn to arguments on behalf of permitting the class of women of reproductive potential to participate in clinical trials, drawing on the ethical principles mentioned above. The first is an argument from justice: the class of men of reproductive potential has never been excluded, although there is evidence that various substances from occupational and pharmaceutical sources affect the male reproductive system. Male-mediated mutagens may include lead, morphine, thalidomide, caffeine, ethanol, and anesthetic gases.[5] Advances in human genetics will surely provide further information about chemical interaction with germ cells in men as well as women. Consistency would therefore require that the class of male subjects of reproductive potential also be rejected. Unless such a "reform" is instituted, debarring the class of women is not only inequitable, it is simply irrational.

One of the defining conditions of a Phase III study is the possibility of benefit for the subject. Thus the exclusion of a class of subjects from clinical trials is a violation of the principle of beneficence toward the potential subjects. On the assumption that information concerning the reaction of women in this age group to a study drug will be beneficial to them, it is also a violation of beneficence toward other women who are not among the subjects.

Worse, therapies are in fact applied to women in this age group in the clinical setting without reliable information concerning hypothetically differential metabolism in this population. Perhaps draconian laws could be established that would discourage such uses of medication by physicians, but this seems both unlikely and impractical. Therefore, exclusionary research policies applied under currently prevailing conditions not only fail to provide some degree of benefit to women of reproductive potential, they are also a source of risk to women.

These considerations establish a *prima facie* case in favor of participation in clinical trials, especially in light of the failure of opposing arguments. I have already alluded to an opposing argument that applies specifically to nonpregnant women, namely, the possibility that they will become pregnant in the course of a trial. As stated, current policies recognize the authority of parents with regard to risks that might be incurred by potential children (fetuses). Therefore I should think that, at most, the same policies would apply with regard to risks that might be incurred with regard to possible children.

This argument does not authorize the prospective subject to accept any and all risk, whether a woman of reproductive potential or a member of any other class. Compounds that do not offer a subject the reasonable prospect of benefits that would offset foreseeable risks should not be brought to a clinical trial. In this context, consider the following scenario: a drug offers a small chance of minor benefit to a subject, but includes a high risk of damage to germ cells. Should such a drug be brought to a clinical trial? I would argue that the harm involved (compromised reproductive well-being) is a harm *to the subject* (male or female), and that the risk–benefit ratio does not justify a clinical trial.

Similarly, participation in Phase I and Phase II studies should be based on an assessment of potential harms to the subject, including damage to her or his reproductive system. Of course, unlike clinical trials, potential benefits to the subject might not be part of such an assessment. However, the presumption of inclusion would place the burden of proof on the argument that the hypothetical risk is unacceptable. Therefore all of the arguments on behalf of participation in clinical trials also apply to studies, except that those that refer to foreseeable benefits to the subject probably would not apply to Phase I studies of toxicity.

On its face, beneficence seems to require the exclusion of women who could become pregnant, but an analysis casts doubt on this inference. Conditions on participation that hinge on a homosexual lifestyle, a promise to avoid pregnancy, or documented sterility would raise daunting problems of verification, would erect decisive obstacles to many worthwhile protocols, and would in many cases have to be applied to men as well as women. Inequitable practices already characterize this area: in trials of a drug (Proscar) that had been found to cause defects in the offspring of male laboratory animals, men were asked only to pledge that they would use "mechanical contraception."[6] The human male's notorious unreliability with respect to such guarantees does not require comment.

I have argued that studies that pose a patently unfavorable balance of risks and benefits should not be offered to women of reproductive age, as they would not be offered to any human subjects; studies that pose no foreseeable risk to the reproductive system should routinely include both male and female subjects. In all other cases, respect for persons implies that individual women of reproductive potential should be the ultimate decision makers with respect to the question whether the risks of participation are acceptable or not. The same ethical principle also requires that subjects understand what they are getting into. Bearing in mind that a consent form should merely document, and not replace, an educational process between the investigator and the candidate, care should be given to ensuring that there is such understanding. Vigorous subject education efforts are indicated when the proposed trial presents a known risk to the reproductive system, in spite of foreseeable benefits to the subject. The intensive "pregnancy prevention program" undertaken by Hoffman-LaRoche, Inc., in connection with the clinical use of Accutane, serves as an example of such initiatives.

In the consent form itself I would recommend language of the following sort:

> It is possible that this treatment will cause damage to children if you choose to have them. You have already been told what is known about this possibility, and you are encouraged to ask further questions. (Include when appropriate: We urge you not to become pregnant while you are part of this study.) You may want to discuss this with others before you agree to take part in this study. If you wish, we will arrange for a doctor, nurse or counselor *who is not part of this study* to discuss this possibility with you and anyone else you want to have present.

This recommendation is consistent with current federal regulations, which require disclosure to subjects of risks that may be incurred by the subject or by the embryo or fetus "if the subject is or may become pregnant. . . ."[7] However, by adopting this language the quoted regulation overlooks male-mediated mutagenesis. When such risks are known prospective male subjects should be engaged in a consent process similar to that described above.

Finally, in our time and in our society, exclusion of a class from participation in a clinical trial has consequences beyond the denial of the specific treatment opportunity.[8] For example, in the area of HIV research there are tangible advantages attached to participation as a research subject for members of the population likely to be at risk, advantages such as improved access to care. In some cases treatment modalities for those who have "failed" with standard medications have only been available within protocol.

In citing these advantages of participation in research for a specific subgroup of women of reproductive age, I open myself to the charge that I am inviting race, sex, and class-based exploitation. Yet it is a canon of research ethics that the benefits as well as the burdens of research should be equitably distributed. Further, the practical implications of exclusion of younger women from clinical trials help to highlight the import of my more general claim, that the class of women of reproductive potential should not be excluded from participation as subjects in research.

Here, then, is a summary of my conclusions:

1. The class of women of reproductive age should be presumed as eligible for enrollment in research.

2. The burden of argument in particular cases should rest on showing that the balance of risks and benefits is patently unacceptable, including harm to the subject's reproductive system without offsetting benefits to the subject.

3. In all other cases the informed consent process should enable the woman to be the ultimate decision maker concerning the acceptability of risks.[9]

An important by-product of these considerations could be a more cautious approach to the investigation and use of drugs in males of reproductive potential.

NOTES

1. Levine, C. 1993. Women as research subjects: New priorities, new questions. In: Emerging Issues in Biomedical Policy: An Annual Review, R.H. Blank and A.L. Bonnicksen, eds. New York: Columbia University Press.

2. Dresser R. Wanted: Single, white male for medical research. *Hastings Center Report* 22(1):24–29.

3. National Commission for the Protection of Human Subjects of Biomedical and Behavioral Research. 1979. The Belmont Report. *Federal Register* 44(76):23192–23197.

4. Levine R. 1986. Ethics and the Regulation of Clinical Research. New Haven: Yale University Press.

5. Soyka, L.F., and Joffe, J.M. 1980. Male-mediated drug effects on offspring. In: Drug and Chemical Risks in the Fetus and Newborn, R.H. Schwartz and S.J. Yaffe, eds. New York: Alan R. Liss. Uzych, L. 1985. Teratogenesis and mutagenesis associated with the exposure of human males to lead: A review. *Yale Journal of Biology*

and Medicine 58:9–17.

6. Comment by Dr. Bonnie Goldmann (Senior Director, Regulatory Affairs, Merck Research Laboratories), Food and Drug Law Institute Conference on Clinical Trials, Washington, D.C., October 5, 1992. Also reported in Debrovner, D. 1993. Of mice and men. *American Druggist* January:30.

7. Department of Health and Human Services. 1983. 45CFR 46.116(b) (1); 21 CFR 50.25(b) (1).

8. Minkoff, H., Moreno, J., and Powderly, P. 1992. Fetal protection and women's access to clinical trials. *Journal of Women's Health* 1:37–41.

9. For their comments on an earlier draft, the author expresses his gratitude to his colleagues in the Division of Humanities in Medicine, and also to Howard Minkoff, M.D., and Richard H. Schwartz, M.D., all of the SUNY Health Science Center at Brooklyn.

Health Consequences of Exclusion or Underrepresentation of Women in Clinical Studies (I)

Carol S. Weisman and Sandra D. Cassard

This paper considers the health consequences to women *as a population* as a result of their exclusion from or underrepresentation in clinical studies. (Clinical studies are broadly defined to include observational studies as well as randomized controlled trials of treatment or preventive interventions). The *reasons* that women, especially women of reproductive age and pregnant women, have been excluded or underrepresented in clinical studies have been amply reviewed.[1] Less apparent are the *consequences* of inadequate studies of women for understanding, preventing, and treating health problems in women. We will describe types of information deficits that exist as a consequence of inadequate research and then examine the evidence of consequences for women's health.

TYPES OF INFORMATION DEFICITS

One type of information deficit occurs for conditions that affect exclusively or primarily women (such as breast cancer and osteoporosis). Failure to conduct sufficient research on these conditions is a special case of exclusion of women from clinical studies and may result in significant gaps in knowledge and in health services for women. If we use as a standard the number of women potentially affected by a condition, then the most obvious information needs pertain to the prevention and treatment of conditions associated with the female reproductive organs and with normal female aging (including menopause). An example of a current information deficit related to aging is the unknown efficacy of estrogen replacement therapy, calcium supplementation, and exercise in preventing osteoporosis and fractures in postmenopausal women.[2]

Another type of information deficit occurs for conditions that affect *both* women and men. These conditions include the leading causes of death in both sexes (cardiovascular disease and lung cancer[3]) as well as conditions that are more prevalent in women (e.g., depression) or that affect men and women differently (e.g., AIDS). Exclusion of women from clinical studies of this class of conditions, or inclusion of women in numbers too small to detect gender differences or to support subgroup analyses, may result in a "male model" of medical treatment that is inappropriate for women.[4] Both biological and psychosocial differences between the sexes may affect etiology, risk factors, disease presentation, disease course, or responses to preventive interventions or treatments. For example, there are numerous information deficits for prevention and treatment of heart disease in women, in part because women were excluded from a number of key trials (e.g., the Lipid Research Clinics Coronary Primary Prevention Trial, the Multiple Risk Factor Intervention Trial, and the Physicians' Health Study). The efficacy of hormone replacement therapy in prevention of heart disease in women is one question requiring further research.[5]

TYPES OF CONSEQUENCES

If there were overall negative health consequences to women as a result of information deficits, we would expect to see them reflected in gender differences in morbidity and mortality; in gender differences in patterns of diagnosis and treatment for key conditions; in gender differences in survival or outcomes of treatments; or in providers' perceptions that their ability to provide optimal care to women patients is compromised. We will examine each of these briefly.

Morbidity and Mortality

Although average life expectancy for U.S. women is about 7 years longer than for men, women consume more health services (including prescription drugs) than men, and throughout life, women experience more disease and disability than men.[6] Further, because women live longer than men, they are more likely to be affected by late-onset diseases such as Alzheimer's disease and osteoporosis.

Mortality trends reveal some interesting gender differences. Although mortality rates from cardiovascular disease have been declining for both sexes over the last two decades, the decline in deaths from ischemic heart disease has been slower for women than for men.[7] In addition, some of the key risk factors for heart disease (e.g., smoking, elevated serum cholesterol, obesity) have not declined as much in women as in men.[8] Reflecting women's smoking patterns, age-adjusted incidence of lung cancer increased steadily from 1980 to 1987 in women, while it did not change substantially for men; death rates parallel the incidence rates.[9] Also owing to smoking patterns, an increase in deaths from chronic obstructive pulmonary disease in women is expected in the next few decades.[10] In 1987, AIDS became the leading cause of death in black women of reproductive age in New York and New Jersey and was expected to be among the five leading causes of death in women in 1991.[11] Among the conditions that are unique to women, breast cancer is the only major cause of mortality.[12] In recent years, breast cancer mortality has increased, especially in black women.[13]

Diagnosis and Treatment Patterns

"Residual exclusion" of women from access to medications tested only on men has been observed in the literature; this occurs when providers are reluctant to use drugs in populations for which safety has not been demonstrated during clinical trials.[14] Other research suggests that women may be diagnosed later or receive less aggressive treatment than men for specific conditions ("referral bias"). Most noteworthy are studies of access among patients with kidney disease to dialysis and transplantation; of diagnosis of lung cancer by sputum cytology; and of diagnosis and treatment of heart disease.[15] Several studies find that women with heart disease may be diagnosed later than men (possibly because tests such as the treadmill exercise test are less effective in women) and that women are less likely than men to have invasive procedures such as coronary angiography, coronary angioplasty, or coronary artery bypass surgery, after relevant covariates such as age and severity are controlled.[16] Although frequently attributed to gender bias in physician decision making, less aggressive treatment also could reflect women patients' beliefs and preferences (although this is undocumented).

Treatment Outcomes

Lower case survival rates have been observed for women following myocardial infarction and diagnosis of AIDS, perhaps reflecting later diagnosis or less aggressive treatment.[17] Another problem is more frequent adverse effects or poorer outcomes for women when drugs or other treatments developed and tested in studies of men are used in women.[18] For example, more women than men appear to experience adverse drug effects, possibly owing to failure to study hormone interactions in drug trials (e.g., for antidepressants).[19]

Higher peri-operative mortality has been observed for women than for men undergoing coronary artery bypass surgery.[20] One possibility is that because of referral bias or difficulties in diagnosis, women receive the procedure at later stages of the disease when their prognosis is poorer. Another possibility is that women's smaller cardiac size or smaller coronary artery diameter may lead to technical problems in surgery. Recent studies report higher mortality for women receiving angioplasty, after controlling for age and severity.[21]

Provider Perceptions

There are no studies of physicians' or other providers' perceptions of whether and to what extent their care of women patients is impeded by the limitations of clinical studies. However, published practice guidelines and consensus reports provide one indicator of whether the professional community recognizes information gaps affecting the treatment of women.

Two recent publications address key risk factors for heart disease, high blood pressure and high serum cholesterol, and both cite gender-related information deficits. The Fifth Report of the Joint National Committee on Detection, Evaluation, and Treatment of High Blood Pressure (JNC V) recommends the same approach to management of hypertension in women and men, although it concludes that further study is warranted and identifies some gaps in knowledge (e.g., effects of hormone replacement therapy on blood pressure).[22] The recommendation for a similar management approach for women and men has been criticized in part because of missing information on the effects of antihypertensive agents on serum lipids in women.[23] With regard to primary prevention of hypertension, however, JNC V does not address gender differences in risk factors (e.g., diet, physical activity, stress levels) or in the efficacy of interventions.[24]

The report of the 1992 NIH Consensus Development Conference on Triglyceride, High-Density Lipoprotein, and Coronary Heart Disease acknowledges information gaps with regard to women and calls specifically for studies of the effects of estrogen and progesterone use on lipids and on risk of coronary heart disease in women.[25]

CONCLUSIONS

Evidence has been provided that exclusion or underrepresentation of women in clinical studies results in some important information deficits, particularly for the leading causes of morbidity and mortality in women, and that these deficits may adversely affect women's health. These deficits, in fact, may result in a shift in the distribution of risks to women in the general population, including pregnant women, who receive treatments (or are impeded from receiving treatments) that have not been developed or studied in women. This transfer of risk from women who are potential participants in clinical studies, where informed consent procedures and monitoring provide safeguards, to women in the general population may be unacceptable as a matter of social policy.

NOTES

1. Institute of Medicine, *Issues in the Inclusion of Women in Clinical Trials,* Washington, DC: National Academy of Sciences, 1991.
2. National Institutes of Health, *Report of the National Institutes of Health: Opportunities for Research on Women's Health,* U.S. Department of Health and Human Services, September 1992.
3. Jacqueline A. Horton (ed.), *The Women's Health Data Book.* Washington, DC: The Jacobs Institute of Women's Health, 1992.
4. Council on Ethical and Judicial Affairs of the American Medical Association, "Gender Disparities in Clinical Decision Making," *JAMA* 266:559–568, 1991.
5. National Women's Health Resource Center, *Forging a Women's Health Research Agenda.* Washington, DC: NWHRC, 1990.
6. NIH, *Opportunities for Research on Women's Health;* Horton (ed.), *The Women's Health Data Book.*
7. Centers for Disease Control, "Trends in Ischemic Heart Disease Mortality—United States, 1980–1988," *MMWR* 41:548, July 31, 1992.
8. NWHRC, *Forging a Women's Health Research Agenda.*
9. Centers for Disease Control, "Trends in Lung Cancer Incidence and Mortality—United States, 1980–1987," *MMWR* 39:875, December 7, 1990.
10. Horton (ed.), *The Women's Health Data Book.*
11. Susan Y. Chu, J. W. Buehler, and Ruth L. Berkelman, "Impact of the Human Immunodeficiency Virus Epidemic on Mortality in Women of Reproductive Age, United States," *JAMA* 264:225–229, 1990.
12. Jeane Ann Grisso and Katherine Watkins, "A Framework for a Women's Health Research Agenda," *Journal of Women's Health* 1:177–183, 1992.
13. Horton (ed.), *The Women's Health Data Book.*
14. Howard Minkoff, Jonathan D. Moreno, and Kathleen R. Powderly, "Fetal Protection and Women's Access to Clinical Trials," *Journal of Women's Health* 1:137–140, 1992.
15. Council Report, "Gender Disparities in Clinical Decision Making," *JAMA* 266:559–562, 1991.
16. John Z. Ayanian and Arnold M. Epstein, "Differences in the Use of Procedures Between Women and Men Hospitalized for Coronary Heart Disease," *NEJM* 325:221–225, 1991; Richard M. Steingart, Milton Packer, Peggy Hamm, et al., "Sex Differences in the Management of Coronary Artery Disease," *NEJM* 325:226–230, 1991; Charles Maynard, Paul E. Litwin, Jenny S. Martin, and Douglas Weaver, "Gender Differences in the Treatment and Outcome of Acute Myocardial Infarction," *Archives of Internal Medicine* 152:972–976, 1992.

17. NIH, *Opportunities for Research on Women's Health;* George F. Lemp, Anne M. Hirozawa, Judith B. Cohen, et al., "Survival for Women and Men with AIDS," *Journal of Infectious Diseases* 166:74–79, 1992.

18. NIH, *Opportunities for Research on Women's Health.*

19. NWHRC, *Forging a Women's Health Research Agenda;* Margaret F. Jensvold, Kathleen Reed, David B. Jarrett, and Jean A. Hamilton, "Menstrual Cycle-Related Depressive Symptoms Treated with Variable Antidepressant Dosage," *Journal of Women's Health* 1:109–115, 1992.

20. Steven S. Khan, Sharon Nessim, Richard Gray, et al., "Increased Mortality of Women in Coronary Artery Bypass Surgery: Evidence for Referral Bias," *Annals of Internal Medicine* 112:561–567, 1990; Edward L. Hannan, Harvey R. Bernard, Harold C. Kilburn, and Joseph F. O'Donnell, "Gender Differences in Mortality Rates for Coronary Artery Bypass Surgery," *American Heart Journal* 123:866–872, 1992.

21. Edward L. Hannan, Djavad T. Arani, Lewis W. Johnson, et al., "Percutaneous Transluminal Coronary Angioplasty in New York State," *JAMA* 268:3092–3097, 1992; Eysmann, Susan B., "Reperfusion and Revascularization Strategies for Coronary Artery Disease in Women," *JAMA* 268:1903–1907, 1992; Sheryl F. Kelsey, Margaret James, Ann Lu Holubkov, et al., "Results of Percutaneous Transluminal Coronary Angioplasty in Women: 1985–1986 National Heart, Lung, and Blood Institute's Coronary Angioplasty Registry," *Circulation* 87:720–727, 1993.

22. Joint National Committee on Detection, Evaluation, and Treatment of High Blood Pressure, "The Fifth Report of the Joint National Committee on Detection, Evaluation, and Treatment of High Blood Pressure (JNC V)," *Archives of Internal Medicine* 153:154–183, 1993.

23. Kathryn Anastos, Pamela Charney, Rita A. Charon, et al., "Hypertension in Women: What is Really Known?" *Archives of Internal Medicine* 115:287–293, 1991.

24. National High Blood Pressure Education Program Working Group, "National High Blood Pressure Education Program Working Group Report on Primary Prevention of Hypertension," *Archives of Internal Medicine* 153:186–208, 1993.

25. National Institutes of Health Consensus Development Panel on Triglyceride, High-Density Lipoprotein, and Coronary Heart Disease, "Triglyceride, High-Density Lipoprotein, and Coronary Heart Disease," *JAMA* 269:505–510, 1993.

Health Consequences of Exclusion or Underrepresentation of Women in Clinical Studies (II)

Leslie Z. Benet

Of course any presentation such as this must begin with the "apple pie" *de rigueur* pronouncement supporting equal access for women in clinical studies. I wholly support such a position and believe that women should be included in all clinical studies in proportion to their prevalence in the population experiencing the phenomena being tested. However, such a position does not address the health consequences of exclusion or underrepresentation. One must, thus, consider separately the Committee's broad definition of the term "clinical studies" to include epidemiological studies, health services research, and outcomes research, as well as randomized clinical trials.

Negative, unacceptable consequences would, and previously did, result from the exclusion or underrepresentation of women in disease epidemiology research, such as the Framingham Study, or in health services research. Similarly, it would be a mistake to exclude women from clinical studies directed toward outcomes research. The latter may be a gray area, since the underrepresentation or exclusion in outcomes research may reflect the lack of clinical investigation where therapeutic interventions are tested. In any case, there seems to be no rationale, except perhaps convention, which could justify the exclusion of women from clinical studies, where no therapeutic intervention is being evaluated.

Therefore, the focus of this presentation will relate to the health consequences of exclusion or underrepresentation of women in randomized clinical trials which involve a therapeutic intervention. Furthermore, let me further exclude the issue of fetal toxicity, as this has been well covered in other presentations. My focus, then, is whether exclusion or underrepresentation underrepresentation of women in clinical studies involving therapeutic interventions may lead to negative health consequences for the potential female population to be administered this therapeutic intervention. Although not all therapeutic interventions will be drugs or chemicals, I will focus my remarks in that area since that is my field.

Basically, the question can be rephrased as, "Will differences in drug disposition or drug response due to gender be clinically significant?" My answer is, "Rarely, if ever."

The basis for my negative response concerning the potential for health consequences in women relates to the intersubject and intrasubject variability which patients exhibit in both the pharmacokinetics and pharmacodynamics of drugs. Most drugs on the market today exhibit a wide therapeutic index. That is, major differences exist between the dose, blood concentration, or receptor concentration necessary to achieve a positive therapeutic response versus those measurements which elicit a toxic response. However, there are a number of drugs critical to our therapeutic armamentarium which exhibit a narrow therapeutic index. That is, small changes in dose or concentration can shift a patient from an efficacious state to a toxic condition or to a state where no efficacy is exhibited (corresponding respectively to increases and decreases in dose or concentration from the therapeutic dosage regimen). It is not well recognized that although many drugs exhibit substantial intrasubject, variability as well as marked intersubject variability, all narrow therapeutic index drugs, by definition, must exhibit low intrasubject variability. If this were not true, a patient maintained on a particular dose would experience cycles of efficacy, lack of efficacy, and toxicity during a constant dosage regimen. In fact, if a narrow therapeutic index drug does exhibit high intrasubject variability, such drugs never get past Phase II testing during the drug development Process, since it is not possible to show efficacy for a particular dose (or steady state concentration).

Narrow therapeutic index drugs, however, may and often do exhibit marked interpatient variability and thus these drugs are titrated in the patient by the clinician to the appropriate dose or concentration, which, once achieved, will be maintained owing to the low intrasubject variability of the drug. It is my hypothesis, that the health consequences of exclusion or underrepresentation of women in clinical studies for narrow therapeutic index drugs will be minimal, since it is immaterial whether women differ significantly from men in their pharmacokinetics and/or pharmacodynamics of the drug, since in each case the drug will be titrated by the clinician to the appropriate dose or concentration.

Similarly, there should be few health consequences to large gender differences for wide therapeutic index or range drugs, since the variability inherent in the male population most likely already encompasses the difference between the male and female patient populations. For the reasons stated above, it seems obvious that we would not have noted any major gender differences in terms of drug kinetics or dynamics for drugs going on the market even though they had received inadequate testing in women. I believe this to be the case.

Although I suspect there are only minimal health consequences of exclusion or underrepresentation of women in clinical studies, I favor inclusion of women as early as possible in drug development, including Phase I studies, but definitely in studies in special populations (e.g., aged, subjects with renal or hepatic disease) and of course in Phase III studies when the treatment will be utilized in women. New techniques in clinical pharmacology, such as population pharmacokinetics, where a few systemic drug concentration measurements are made in each patient during Phase III, can be utilized to identify the presence or lack of drug–drug and drug–disease interactions, and to identify other unanticipated variabilities such as metabolic heterogeneity, as well as gender differences. Such information will be useful in understanding the drug disposition process as a function of gender, age, disease, environment, and chronopharmacologic effects.

An example of such a gender dependent finding relates to the explosion of knowledge about drug metabolizing isozymes which has occurred during the last few years. We have identified, purified, characterized, and cloned specific isozymes with emphasis on the major metabolic system—the cytochromes P450. At least seven, and maybe more, gene superfamilies have been identified in humans. Furthermore, innumerable isozymes of the cytochromes P450 and other enzyme systems are continuing to be identified, both in humans and in the animal species used in preclinical testing. Up until now, no marked gender difference in the presence of these isozymes has been identified in humans, although certain animal species do exhibit marked gender specific differences in various isozyme levels. In one case, for a very important human metabolic isozyme, identified as P450-3A4, a potential gender difference has been suggested. Earlier this week at the National Institutes of Health's "Workshop on Menopause," I hypothesized that clearance in postmenopausal women is lower than that in premenopausal women for many drugs owing to the decrease of a particular metabolic isozyme. I suggested that the isozyme which is decreased in menopause is P450-3A4. I further hypothesized that progestational agents may restore P450-3A4 to pre-menopausal levels. If my hypotheses are correct, then a gender difference due to menopause, which previously may have been confounded with an age effect, could be important in evaluating and optimizing new drug therapies, as well as in correctly defining the disposition of drugs in postmenopausal women not receiving progestational agents. The hypotheses which I made could only be developed as a result of our increasing understanding of the importance and specificity of the metabolic isozymes. But, the results above could not be obtained if studies were not carried out comparing pre- and postmenopausal women.

Therefore, in conclusion, although I feel that there are minimal immediate health consequences to the exclusion or underrepresentation of women in clinical studies, the advancement of therapy and our understanding of the basic processes involved can only be enhanced by inclusion of women at all levels of clinical investigation.

Recruitment and Retention of Women in Clinical Studies: Theoretical Perspectives and Methodological Considerations

Diane B. Stoy

Recruiting and retaining subjects in clinical studies are challenging tasks that are critical to the success of any study. Recent federal regulations regarding the inclusion of women in clinical studies have sparked new interest in (1) defining gender differences relevant to the recruitment and retention of subjects in clinical studies, and (2) developing gender-specific recruitment and retention strategies. This paper presents an overview of relevant differences between men and women, the implications of these differences for recruitment and retention, and some practical considerations for researchers conducting studies with female subjects.

THE DYNAMICS OF RECRUITMENT AND RETENTION

In clinical studies, the assessment of recruitment and retention is typically reported with quantitative measures such as the number of subjects screened for a study, the yield from specific recruitment sources, the subjects' adherence to a schedule of clinic visits, and the subjects' adherence to a regimen with an investigational medication. In reality, such quantitative measures reflect a social process of interaction between researchers and their subjects. Any discussion of recruitment or retention, therefore, must begin with the broad social context in which researchers and subjects develop their unique relationship.

The interaction begins with the first contact between a potential subject and the researchers. This contact may be sparked by the subject's attraction to the

45

potential personal benefits derived from participating in a study and/or a study's appeal to the subject's altruism or affiliation needs. The interaction between researcher and participant then continues with the informed consent process in which the study design, risks, benefits, alternatives, researcher's responsibilities, and extent of the participant commitment are reviewed. Throughout the study's data collection phase, subjects fulfill their commitment to the researchers and the study protocol by performing a variety of specified behavioral tasks such as visiting the clinical center regularly for health assessments, completing health questionnaires, following a diet, or taking medication. Thus, the processes of recruitment and retention involve the mutual participation of researchers and study subjects in the implementation of a study protocol; an agreement between the researchers and the subjects about the behaviors required for that implementation; and the performance of those behaviors within the social context of the subjects' lives.

Are there gender differences that affect the way in which women versus men perceive participation in clinical studies? Experience in clinical research suggests that there are differences, and that these differences are not only grounded in biology but also profoundly shaped by culture and patterns of human development.

CROSS-CULTURAL DIFFERENCES: MEN VS. WOMEN

Since the days of Freud, the differences between men and women have been the subject of great debate, the full extent of which is beyond the scope of this paper. It is safe to say that until recently, analytic approaches in the social sciences have relied on the male model as the gold standard, and have not been told from a feminine perspective.

Despite this bias toward men, there is a general recognition across social science disciplines of distinct differences between men and women that extend beyond biology. According to Williams (1987), "the values and interests of females collectively are different in important, measurable ways from those of males in this society" (p. 190). These differences stem from the fact that men and women are socialized differently into two distinct cultures: manhood and womanhood. Although considerable geographic, generational, economic, religious, and ethnic variations exist, there is a constellation of gender-specific values, beliefs, and cultural imperatives. These values, beliefs, and imperatives—in conjunction with biological differences—represent the intersection of culture and biology, and have implications for the recruitment and retention of female subjects.

According to psychologists (Williams, 1987; Miller, 1986; Johnson and Ferguson, 1990) the lives of contemporary women, like those of generations before them—are organized around "giving" to and serving others, and it is from this dynamic that women derive a major part of their self-worth. As the bearers and primary caretakers of children, women typically submerge their own personality and subjugate their own needs to those of their families. Miller (1986) suggests that many of contemporary women's activities are undertaken in pursuit not of their own goals, but of the goals of others such as their spouse and children. Women's sense of self is also organized around being able to maintain affiliations and relationships with others.

Activities directed at achieving personal goals, says Miller, can "easily be fraught with conflict and can contribute to diminishing a woman's self-image" (p. 54). The role conflict of contemporary women, i.e, the balancing of career and family needs, can result in "being pulled in all directions" (Williams, 1987, p. 299) and in the superwoman syndrome, in which women suffer exhaustion as they struggle to satisfy their family, career, and personal needs.

In contrast, Miller (1986) suggests that men's lives—with their focus on "doing"—are psychologically organized against the principle of giving to others. Men's images revolve around selfseeking achievement and competition, the hallmarks that characterize the male culture. According to Miller, serving others is a "luxury a man desires or can afford only after he has fulfilled the primary requirements of manhood. Once he has become a man by other standards, he may choose to serve others" (p. 70). In his pivotal work on human development, Erickson (1968) used the male experience as the model for his eight progressive stages of the development of "man." These stages, said Erickson, are those that individuals must pass through on the path to maturity. Erickson postulated that, for women, intimacy preceded identity, and that a woman was expected to subjugate her aspirations to those of her husband and to the care of him and their children. Erickson also insisted that female psychology was driven by biology, and that a woman's identity was derived from her reproductive role. Erickson has been criticized (Johnson and Ferguson, 1990) for failing to recognize the developmental impact of sex roles and the limitations that role expectations placed on women's equal participation in society.

The work of Erickson (1968) as well as that of Levinson (1978) and Vaillant (1978) extended the study of human development past adolescence to the entire life span. The concept that psychological growth and development continued from birth until death was later popularized by Sheehy in her book *Passages*, although Sheehy and her colleagues in human development have been criticized for extrapolating the data from the study of men to women.

Contemporary views of life span theory suggest that the sequence and intensity of the predictable life stages of adults are truly different in men and women, even in today's society in which women have gained fuller participation. These differences arise from the impact of childbearing and parenting, which remain female functions, and social changes, such as improved occupational mobility, which arose from the woman's movement. Although there is always individual variation within cultural groups, these differences can generally be seen in the life patterns of men and women today. The life development pattern for men in early and middle adulthood is primarily focused on career achievement, with parenting generally relegated to a secondary role. After the attainment of career goals in mid-life, men's primary focus is thought to shift away from career issues and toward the enrichment of relationships with family and community.

Conversely, in early adulthood, the lives of women revolve primarily around their parenting responsibilities, which often take precedence over their career aspirations. Contrary to popular belief, studies of women with an "empty nest" suggest that women experience mid-life differently than men. Free from the parenting responsibilities of small children, women at mid-life are finally free to satisfy their individual needs for achievement by focusing their energies on their own career aspirations. Thus, the life pattern of women and men at early and middle adulthood appears to be remarkably different.

GENDER DIFFERENCES: IMPLICATIONS FOR RESEARCH

Scientific evidence and clinical experience suggest that there may be significant differences in the recruitment and retention of male and female subjects. For example, as the primary caretaker of children, a young woman with a family may be hesitant to enroll in a study that presents potential risks to her safety and livelihood, and ultimately that of her children. A working mother may also be hesitant to participate because she may be unable to incorporate the behavioral requirements of the study into her daily schedule in which she already experiences stress from conflicting role demands.

For example, a young mother may wish to reserve her annual or sick leave for the days when her children are ill, rather than a half or whole day of study-related health assessments. Women who agree to participate in a study may also experience some life crises in her family, such as a serious illness of a child, that may limit her short- and long-term ability to conform to the requirements of a study protocol.

There are also generational differences among women that are important to acknowledge. For example, women over the age of 65—who did not grow up in the era of self-help, preventive medicine, or communal exercise such as aerobic dancing—may be less willing to participate in studies that conflict with their prevailing beliefs about health. These beliefs may include such ideas as not taking hormone replacement because they feel well and believe that "if it's not broken, don't fix it"; or not participating in a study involving group exercise because they feel uncomfortable undressing and exercising with strangers. Women in this age group also may be unwilling to agree to participate in a study without discussing the study with their spouse or family.

There are also special considerations for older women related to aging, social roles, and cultural biases. For example, one recruitment campaign for a clinical study of postmenopausal estrogen replacement was a dismal failure in metropolitan Washington, D.C., when it was advertised by the media as a "menopause" study. Focus groups later revealed that the failure of the recruitment was directly related to the use of the word "menopause" in the advertising. In the youth-oriented American society, menopause is synonymous with aging, which has negative connotations for women. Thus, women were hesitant to be associated with a study of aging women. The same type of study, however, later enjoyed an enormously successful recruitment campaign when the study's recruitment director eliminated the word menopause from its publicity materials and instead used "Women have hearts, too!" as the study's theme.

Another consideration is the difference between men and women in the age of onset of disease. Studies of women with heart disease, for example, involve women who are generally 10 to 20 years older than their male peers with heart disease. These older women are often less independent and less mobile. This lack of independence can be a considerable barrier to participation in a study that involves regular visits to a clinical center. Even in an urban area such as metropolitan Washington, D.C., many older women do not have a driver's license or are unwilling to drive into the city. In addition, once enrolled in a study, older women such as these with a variety of medical problems are often unwilling to travel to the center in inclement weather. For example, on a recent rainy Friday afternoon in Washington, D.C., all five women who were scheduled to visit the clinical center for an introductory visit did not keep their appointments as scheduled. Although concerns about mobility are evidenced in older men and women, the fact that heart disease manifests itself at a later age in women increases the recruitment and retention difficulties inherent in heart disease studies in women.

METHODOLOGICAL CONSIDERATIONS FOR RESEARCHERS

What actions can researchers take to assure the full participation of women in clinical studies? The starting point, I believe, is to acknowledge that there *are* distinct differences between men and women. Although there are always variations within and across groups, there are distinct biological, cultural, and developmental differences between men and women that can directly and indirectly affect women's participation in clinical research.

Given these differences, researchers who are conducting studies with women may consider the following:

1. *Providing young women with children and older women with very*

specific and clear information about the behavioral requirements of the study. Since a selective recruitment process can enhance long-term retention, researchers should make every effort during the consent process to clarify the behavioral requirements of the study. Although this information must be reviewed as part of the informed consent, it often becomes lost among the myriad of details in the consent form. Therefore, it is helpful to provide participants with a separate document that clearly outlines the study's visit schedule, the procedures required at each visit, and the time required for each. This document should also specify what time of day the clinic visits must occur (early/late morning, afternoons or evenings), the locations to which the subjects must report, and how flexible the scheduling can be. For example, in one multicenter study of postmenopausal hormone replacement, the subjects were required to spend one full day and one half day a year undergoing health assessments such as blood clotting studies, endometrial biopsies, and mammography. Other studies may involve regular blood testing or urine collection throughout the work day, or admission to a metabolic unit in a hospital.

2. *Offering flexible scheduling and child care.* Women with young children may be willing to participate in clinical studies if they can complete their clinic visits during school hours, or if the clinical center will provide short-term child care. Some interested women may be willing to participate if the clinical center offers evening and Saturday appointments. Flexible scheduling is also important for women who are faced with a family crisis that they must handle in addition to their other roles. Researchers may be able to obtain administrative leave for their study subjects by writing a letter to the subject's supervisor.

3. *Offering assistance with transportation.* Both older and younger women who do not drive may require assistance with local transportation. Some universities provide door-to-door van transportation, while others provide reimbursement for taxicabs, bus transportation, or local parking.

4. *Allowing extra time to carefully review the study's risks and benefits with female subjects.* Although women are socialized into a giving role, they may be hesitant to participate in a study in which there are considerable risks. Adequate time should be spent discussing the risks and benefits with the woman, and if desired, with her significant other. Sending the study materials home in advance of the clinic visit is helpful because it gives a woman time to review the materials in the privacy of her home before returning to the clinical center.

5. *Designing the recruitment materials for the study in a way that is sensitive to women.* This means careful wording of references to age, sexuality, fertility, menopausal symptoms, etc. It is helpful to enlist the services of public relations professionals with experience in women's health. In addition, the use of focus groups is a cost effective method for test marketing preliminary recruitment aterials and identifying potential problems with recruitment materials.

6. *Making every effort to recognize the women's contribution to the research effort.* The multiple and often conflicting roles of contemporary women leave women with little spare time. Women who participate in clinical studies, who have given their time and energy, should be recognized for their contribution. This may be done with special study-sponsored events, certificates of appreciation, study-related memorabilia, etc.

REFERENCES

Erickson, E. (1968) *Identity: Youth and Crisis.* New York: W. W. Norton & Company, Inc.

Levinson, D. J. (1978) *The Season's of a Man's Life.* New York: Ballantine.

Miller, J. B. (1986) *Toward a New Psychology of Women.* Boston: Beacon Press.

Johnson, K., and T. Ferguson. (1990) *Trusting Ourselves: The Sourcebook on Psychology for Women.* New York: Atlantic Monthly Press.

Vaillant, G. E. (1978) *Adaptation to Life.* Boston: Little, Brown.

Williams, J. H. (1987) *Psychology of Women: Behavior in a Biosocial Context.* New York: W. W. Norton & Company, Inc.

Recruitment and Retention of Women of Color in Clinical Studies

Janet L. Mitchell

The focus on the underrepresentation of women of color in clinical studies has benefitted from the scrutiny of the underrepresentation of women and minorities in AIDS research and recent public attention highlighting the practice of routinely excluding *all* women from certain studies. While others will discuss the reasons for the exclusion of women as a whole, minority status and economic circumstance represent unique aspects that need to be addressed separately.

Before one begins to discuss these issues, it is important to examine a few fundamental questions. The focus on the exclusion of women from clinical studies has as its basis *rejection* of the concept that men or "maleness" is the norm and that women are fundamentally no different from men and therefore findings in male subjects can be generalized to all persons whether male or female. Since until very recently men—white men—dominated the research field, including the setting of priorities, it stands to reason that they would view themselves as the standard. Although the numbers of women in the research arena have been increasing, again the increase has been basically "white women." It is important to examime how research "norms" are then defined. In fact, is important to examine how society defines itself and all "norms," if one is to critically focus on issues related to people of color and by extension women of color. While those parties concerned with the exclusion of women from clinical studies are quite willing to recognize the premise of men being the standard as flawed, they are less willing to consider the possibility that defining society and norms on the basis of white Anglo- or Euro-centric beliefs may also be flawed. This country is not the melting pot that many would like to believe it is and, in fact, it is comprised of many diverse cultures, races, and ethnicities—all of which have the same right to define society and norms from

52

their own unique perspective. It is this premise that allows for the following perspective on the underrepresentation of women of color in clinical studies.

Although it is important to understand that women of color are a very heterogeneous group, as are all groups, certain historical experiences are common and account for certain attitudes and perceptions.

Distrust of the "intent" of the white community can be found at all educational and economical levels. While many are aware of the Black Power movement of the 1960s and 1970s, there is a similar movement today that is less visible to the white community but is well-known in the African American community. It is described by the adjective "Afro-centric" but has a philosophy rooted in distrust of anything that is "Euro-centric"; calls for self-reliance and self-determination. The medical community encountered the movement in the controversy around Kemron.* The perception that Kemron was a treatment developed by an African and the belief, again regardless of educational or economic status, that the virus that causes AIDS may be man-made has as much to do with the underrepresentation of minorities in AIDS clinical studies as does the circumstance of gender, economics, or drug use.

A review of the literature on the recruitment of minorities into clinical studies revealed that authors are more comfortable discussing issues that related to economic and institutional barriers than they are discussing attitudinal barriers. This is even true of the one recent article that addresses, in a real way, most of the barriers encountered when recruiting and retaining minorities in clinical studies. I refer you to the article written by two colleagues at Harlem Hospital Center, who at that time were responsible for the NIH-/NIAID-funded Community Program for Clinical Research on AIDS (CPCRA), entitled "The Challenge of Minority Recruitment in Clinical Trials for AIDS."[1] This is by far the most comprehensive discussion of many of the barriers to minority recruitment and retention with recommendations that would be endorsed by anyone who has ever worked with this population. However, while mentioning the distrust of the community and citing the Tuskegee experiment, the authors chose to focus on economic barriers. They also chose to focus on the idea that the underrepresentation of minorities in studies can lead to confusion in

---

*Kemron is the trade name for a drug, alpha interferon, discovered by an American but first used in AIDS patients by a researcher from Kenya, Davy Koech. Koech reported that AIDS patients taking the drug improved remarkably; however, the U.S. scientific community dismissed his claims as based on small, uncontrolled studies. There were protests from the African American community that the white, U.S. scientific establishment had rejected a promising African innovation (Cowley, G., "The Angry Politics of Kemron," *Newsweek,* Jan. 4, 1993, 43–44). Although both NIAID and the WHO have now refuted Koech's claims, NIH has begun clinical trials of Kemron in the United States (F-D-C Reports, Inc., *The Blue Sheet,* June 9, 1993, 12). — Ed.

interpretation. Just as there can be gender-specific differences in response to treatment, there can also be racial/ethnic differences as has been demonstrated in racial differences in response to antihypertension therapy. The authors lead one to believe that the refusal of many of their patients to take zidovudine (AZT) was due to the result of one study that concluded that the drug may not benefit African Americans or Latinos. What my colleagues failed to mention was that even before the release of that study, African Americans did not truly believe that the drug was of benefit. The release of the study only gave them the scientific ammunition needed to confront the medical establishment. As committed and dedicated as my colleagues are, and they are, they are neither African American nor Latina. Therefore they share the same discomfort as many in the white community of not wanting to confront issues that highlight the inherent racism in this country, even in medicine.

One other article that examined psychosocial influences on recruitment and retention of women attending a family planning clinic did not look at these differences across races despite the fact that the study includes 4,781 women—18 percent of whom were African American.[2]

Another historical experience that cuts across all educational and economic levels in communities of color, which can be perceived as a barrier to recruitment and retention, is that of spirituality. "I will leave it in God's (Allah's) hands" is an expression medical providers hear often from their patients of color. Spirituality is seen as a major cornerstone in the foundation for survival. It is especially called upon when one is faced with life-and-death crises, such as a terminal illness. Many providers, regardless of color, have learned to use that spirituality to the benefit of science by making it a partner. "It is God (Allah) that helped me become a physician (nurse, etc.)." "It was God (Allah) that enabled the treatment to be developed." Communities of color are less enamored with traditional science and technology. The reliance on spirituality and alternative treatments, often as the *first* choice in communities of color, is now recognized and being viewed less negatively by traditional science, as evidenced by the establishment at the National Institutes of Health of an Office on Alternative Therapies. One paper that looked at recruitment strategies for multiethnic families found the use of religious associations and their leaders as purveyors of the message more effective in recruiting African American families for participation than media, posters, and telephone contacts.[3]

What is often not seen as a barrier but can be a significant deterrent in communities of color is the time involved in participation in clinical studies. This barrier can be related to loss of income or lack of time. While there is a growing middle class in communities of color, there is still a gap in the earning potential and job status. The middle class status of many families is dependent on two incomes or multiple jobs. The job position may not allow for much flexibility. This translates for many into loss of income for the time needed for follow-up or the inability to find the time for follow-up because of multiple responsibilities.

While these first three issues are generic to communities of color in general, women of color have specific issues that may be viewed as barriers in recruitment and retention into clinical studies. Again, regardless of educational or economic status, women of color are more accepting of the traditional roles of women as caregivers and caretakers. The statistics that highlight the large number of single-female-headed households in communities of color lead to false assumptions about the role and philosophy of that single female. Some would like to believe that that status has brought her closer to a philosophy of taking care of self first. In reality, most women of color are single by circumstances, not by choice. Despite that status of "single female head of (one) household," at any given time they are responsible in a very traditional sense for their own children (if they are mothers), other children in the family, other members of their family, their partner (be that male or female), or a neighbor. Whether employed outside the home or not, women of color still bear the primary responsibility of providing sustenance, comfort, and support. This can be in any combination—financial, spiritual, moral, and/or physical. All of this leads to their putting the needs of others before their own. Using the example of AIDS again, successful programs targeted to women recognized the importance of providing care for children (infected or not) in conjunction with care for their mothers. Some programs have also extended this to partners. All programs know that when asked about missed appointments, women often report needing to attend to the needs of some other person. Because this traditional role extends to providers, women of color, especially those less well educated or less well-off economically are reluctant to admit that there may be a conflict of time or philosophy. This is especially true if there was no initial discussion that allowed the woman to feel she was a partner in the process and that her opinion was important.

Because of this traditional role (often interpreted as passivity) and the historical exploitation of this population by medicine, many have concerns about their vulnerability to coercion. Unfortunately, the potential for this still exists, despite the existence of institutional review boards. It is important to again view this from a historical perspective. Just as spirituality has been a cornerstone in the foundation of survival of communities of color, so too has sacrifice. The incentives that most clinical studies are beginning to offer for participation may be of more importance from the perspective of the participant than the study intended. This is especially true for parents (mothers). The offer of disposable diapers, cribs, and strollers may be the overriding reason for participation. While this is a concern and should be considered when including incentives, it is also important to understand that communities of color are much less trusting and in fact quite suspicious still of "research." While reasons to participate or not may differ from that of the white community, the reasons are usually just as sound, albeit from a different cultural context.

It is important to understand that there is often a direct link to the "lost to follow-up" and the perception of coercion. If the perception is that care and service depends upon participation in a clinical study in which one does not want to participate, one goes elsewhere. Be careful as to how data on this population have been interpreted in the past. The use of the emergency room and episodic care has as much to do with the attitude of the clinic staff (especially the clerk), the ability to be seen by the same provider, and the flexibility of the clinic's hours, as do the complexities in the individual's life. Given the fiscal situation in most publicly run facilities, this will only get worse.

Across all educational and economic strata the numbers of women of color enrolled in clinical studies are low. Attempts to analyze this phenomenon have focused mainly on low-income women of color. The identification of many barriers such as transportation, child care, language, etc., are well documented. Even the element of distrust is noted. Yet numbers are low for educated, higher-income women as well. This issue has received less attention. In this group the attitudinal barriers may dominate. There are also institutional barriers that have not been given enough importance. To answer the question of how to increase the participation of women of color in clinical studies, we must first revisit an assumption. I suggest we first seek answers to the following questions from a representative sample across all educational and economic levels:

1. Do women of color feel that participation in clinical studies is important? Why or why not?

2. Do women of color feel that *their* participation is important? Why or why not?

3. For women who were offered an opportunity to participate but declined, why?

4. For women who were not offered an opportunity to participate, why do you feel you were not offered the opportunity? For the provider, why was the opportunity not offered?

NOTES

1. El-Sadr, W., and Capps, L. 1992. Special communication: The challenge of minority recruitment in clinical trials for AIDS. *Journal of the American Medical Association* 267:954–957.

2. Young, C. L., and Dombrowski, M. 1989. Psychosocial influences on research subject recruitment, enrollment and retention. *Social Work in Health Care* 14:43–57.

3. Hooks, P.C., Tsong, Y., Baranowski, T., et al. 1988. Recruitment strategies for multiethnic family and community health research. *Family and Community Health* 11:48–59.

Recruitment and Retention of Women in Clinical Studies: Ethical Considerations

Robert J. Levine

INCENTIVES TO ENROLL AND TO CONTINUE PARTICIPATION

The first principle of the Nuremberg Code reads, in part: ". . . the person . . . should be so situated as to be able to exercise *free power of choice*, without the intervention of any element of force, fraud, deceit, duress, overreaching, or other ulterior form of constraint or coercion. . . ."

Of primary concern is that incentives offered to prospective subjects may be so great as to become an "ulterior form of constraint" which will overcome or overwhelm the individual's capacity to exercise free power of choice; such incentives are commonly called "undue inducements."

In the literature on inducements or incentives, some are usually considered unproblematic. These include (1) altruism; (2) reimbursement for out-of-pocket expenses such as transportation and daycare; and (3) free investigational drugs and other medical goods and services.

There are some who consider the problem of reimbursements more difficult or complicated for women than it is for men. Women are more likely (so it is argued) to require transportation, babysitters, daycare, and other services for which reimbursements are required. In this regard it is worth noticing that men may also require reimbursements for daycare, transportation, and babysitters.

In my view, reimbursements for out-of-pocket expenses are ethically unproblematic. They do not represent constraints in that the recipients do no better than break even; financially, their position is neither improved nor diminished.

Free investigational drugs and other medical goods and services, although usually considered ethically unproblematic, may be much more powerful inducements than cash payments. The value of free medical goods and services can be overwhelming, particularly for poor people. This is equally true for men and women.

Cash payments are usually considered at least potentially problematic even though their actual value may be substantially less than that of free medical goods and services.

In order to gain some perspective on this issue, let us consider a protocol that was approved by several institutional review boards (IRBs). The protocol consisted of a placebo-controlled, randomized clinical trial of a new "me-too" antihypertensive drug. The subjects were called upon to go through a 2-week "placebo-washout" period followed by 26 weeks of taking either active drug or placebo. Subjects were to be paid $1500 at the conclusion of the trial. In addition, they were to receive free "drug" and free clinic visits each week.

This case is not atypical; many clinical trials offer similar inducements and they are customarily approved by IRBs. I want to make two general points about the inducements in this protocol. Firstly, the inducements offered to participate in this clinical trial make our arguments about the propriety of reimbursing subjects for out-of-pocket expenses seem rather trivial. Secondly, it must be acknowledged that the purpose of this payment is to induce prospective subjects to do what they would not otherwise do. There is nothing necessarily problematic about this. All of us are paid to do things that we would not otherwise do. Payments become problematic only when they might overwhelm a prospective subject's judgment about whether she or he wishes to participate.

In general, IRBs do not seem to worry very much about cash payments or other material inducements in situations in which the risk is acceptably low or in which the risks appear to be in reasonable proportion to the anticipated direct health-related benefits to the subject. In such cases, there is a tendency to let market factors determine the amount of payments. By contrast, where the risk is high and there is no reasonable expectation of proportionately high direct health-related benefits to subjects, IRBs tend to aspire to the ideal of altruism by keeping payments low.

In the category of incentives to enroll or to continue participation, I am not aware of any considerations that apply peculiarly to women that do not apply equally to men.

FREE ABORTION AS AN INCENTIVE

One of the reasons that women are often excluded from clinical trials of new drugs is concern that during the course of the clinical trial they might become pregnant and that the fetus could be deformed. In short, there is great anxiety about repeating the thalidomide experience.

This raises some questions: Is it permissible for a sponsor to offer a free abortion to women who become pregnant? If so, is it permissible to exclude women who would not freely choose to have an abortion if they became pregnant during the course of a clinical trial?

I believe that our responses to such questions must take into account several features of the clinical trial. Following are attributes of clinical trials listed in descending order of their providing ethical justification for responding "yes" to one or both of the two questions. (In general, the justification for responding "yes" to the second question must be stronger than that required for a "yes" response to the first question.)

1. The purpose of the clinical trial is to evaluate a new contraceptive or contragestive agent. That is, the subjects enrolled with the expectation that they would avoid or terminate pregnancy.

2. The agent being evaluated is known to be teratogenic in humans.

3. Preclinical tests of the agent being evaluated suggest that it might be teratogenic in humans.

4. Preclinical tests for mutagenicity and teratogenicity have not been done.

5. Preclinical tests show no evidence of mutagenicity or teratogenicity.

But what, one might ask, if a drug known to be teratogenic in humans offers the only possible means of arresting or delaying the progress of a lethal or disabling disease and a woman, fully informed of the risks, says she wants the drug, but cannot accept abortion as a matter of conscience. I would make it available to her if she agreed to use a highly effective means of contraception and if she agreed to assume all of the burdens of giving birth to an impaired child, should that occur. In other words, I do not believe coerced abortion can be justified. (Even if a woman agreed to assume all of the burdens of giving birth to an impaired child, I would not hold the child accountable for such a decision. Such a child should be offered financial assistance as necessary for any special needs [e.g., special education] he or she might have as a consequence of the impairment.)

DEALING WITH DROPOUTS

The passage in Department of Health and Human Services regulations that speaks to this issue is Section 46.116(a)(8) of Title 45 of the Code of Federal Regulations: ". . . in seeking informed consent the following information shall be provided to each subject. . . . A statement that participation is voluntary . . . and the subject may discontinue participation at any time without penalty or loss of benefits to which the subject is otherwise entitled."

The philosopher Lisa Newton argues that the completely unfettered freedom to withdraw which is required by ethical codes and regulations "is an anomaly in ethics, since it appears to be . . . in direct conflict with [one's] ordinary duty to keep [one's] promises" (Newton, 1984). She recommends that future formulations of regulations should recognize that the relationship between researcher and subject is "binding on both sides, hence to be taken very seriously on both sides, and go on to specify the circumstances that shall be taken to negate or cancel that mutual commitment."

IRBs seem to be acting as if they partially agree with Newton as they routinely approve plans to withhold part or all of cash payments from subjects who withdraw without having some plausible excuse such as an adverse reaction to a drug.

What about "quiet dropouts"—those who simply miss appointments without ever asserting their right to withdraw without penalty? Is it permissible to contact them (e.g., by repeated telephone calls) to try to persuade them to return?

The answer, I believe, is "yes." I believe that it is important to anticipate such behaviors in the informed consent process. Prospective subjects should be made aware of plans to contact them because some may consider such attempts unwelcome intrusions or threats to their privacy.

In some clinical trials such plans have been rather elaborate. For example, in the Multiple Risk Factor Intervention Trial protocol, the investigators enlisted the aid of an investigative services firm in locating subjects with whom they had lost contact for 12 months or more. After attempts to locate the subjects through "local resources and Social Security" failed, they provided the investigative services firm with the subject's name, last known address and telephone number, place of employment and work phone, and names and addresses of persons indicated by the subject as those likely to know his whereabouts. These procedures were publicized widely without adverse criticism.

Some commentators have expressed concern that women may be "less empowered" by their nature to assert their rights to withdraw from research, particularly given their greater (than men's) proclivities to value and maintain relationships. This could be problematic in some types of clinical research. This is a potential problem that should be called to the attention of IRBs and investigators.

I would like to call attention to another likely problem—that in some randomized clinical trials women might be inclined to either drop out or engage in covert noncompliance. Let us consider, for example, the Breast Cancer Prevention Trial (BCPT), a placebo-controlled trial of tamoxifen for the prevention of breast cancer. Newspapers around the country have popularized the debate over the so-called "serious" adverse effects of tamoxifen such as induction of cancer or life-threatening liver damage. But they have reported little or nothing about the so-called "minor" side effects which, in my view, are much more likely to undermine the validity of BCPT.

Tamoxifen, in the dose prescribed in BCPT, produces a relatively high rate of unpleasant side effects such as vaginal dryness and hot flashes. Many women may reconsider their commitment to endure such discomforts a full 5 years, particularly if they recall and believe the statements made to them during the informed consent process about the initial null hypothesis or state of "clinical equipoise" that justified beginning the randomized clinical trial. One such woman might ask, "Does it make sense for me to put up with hot flashes and vaginal dryness for 5 years when the doctors say that tamoxifen is not known to be more or less beneficial than placebo which, in turn, is the same as nothing?" If she decides that it does not make sense, she may either drop out of the trial or engage in covert noncompliance, skipping some or most of her doses of tamoxifen.

But, one might ask, is that not what the process of informed consent is designed to prevent? Can we not anticipate that women who are unwilling to accept a chance of these symptoms will refuse to enroll in the study? Some will, of course, but there is a great difference between the acceptance of a statistical chance of the occurrence of symptoms by a women who has never experienced them and the subsequent lived reality of hot flashes and vaginal dryness.

If there is a high rate of dropouts or covert noncompliance, this will seriously undermine the validity of this clinical trial. Perhaps this should alert us to the need to involve in the design of such clinical trials people who are sensitive to such possibilities.

COSTS OF INVOLVING WOMEN AS RESEARCH SUBJECTS

Some sponsors of research, both industrial and governmental, have claimed that inclusion of women as research subjects raises the costs of doing research to the extent that their exclusion is justified on ethical grounds. Such sponsors hold that there is an unacceptably high cost–benefit ratio.

One cannot deny categorically the validity of cost–benefit considerations in determining whether certain research projects should be done. There are some interesting bits of knowledge that are simply not worth the expense of their acquisition. In general, however, I would deny the validity of such considerations as a justification for excluding women from most research projects.

Women have been excluded from studies of new drugs owing to concern that there might be damage to their fetuses should they become pregnant. One cannot deny the validity of this concern. As a partial response to this concern, I favor the development of no-fault compensation systems for injured research subjects. This does not mitigate the grief of bearing or being a handicapped child. It would, however, relieve the at-times overwhelming financial consequences for both sponsors and subjects.

It is very unlikely that we will ever see another "thalidomide." Tests that would have detected the problem caused by thalidomide are now done routinely in the preclinical phase of drug development. But let us consider a hypothetical case. Consider a new drug that, like thalidomide, caused a severe congenital anomaly by a mechanism that could not be detected by preclinical testing. Let us further assume that, like thalidomide, the anomaly it caused also occurred "naturally" in a small percentage of babies whose mothers did not take the new drug.

If the first administration of this drug to women who could and did become pregnant were conducted in the context of a carefully monitored clinical trial, the association between the drug and the anomaly could be detected after the occurrence of only a small number of anomalies. If instead, the first administration of this drug to women who could and did become pregnant took place in the relatively unmonitored context of clinical practice, then, as with thalidomide, the association between the drug and the anomaly would not be established until hundreds or thousands of babies were born with the anomaly. As with thalidomide, each obstetrician would believe the anomaly she or he observed was one of the unusual cases that occurred "naturally."

Women also are excluded from "basic research" designed not to develop drugs but rather to understand basic physiological processes. They are excluded because phasic variations in their physiological processes make such research difficult and more costly. It is more costly because larger numbers of subjects must be studied. Such exclusion is also unjust. Women are entitled to have basic information about their physiological processes studied and understood. The "norms" established by doing research on men should no longer be considered *the normal*. Data derived from studies of healthy women also reflect a normality, albeit, in some cases, a more complicated normality. Moreover, such studies often become the bases for subsequent development of diagnostic, prophylactic, and therapeutic products.

TWO SEPARATE AGENDAS ON THE INCLUSION OF WOMEN

Considerations of distributive justice provide the ethical grounding for arguments that women ought to be included as subjects in research. I want to point out that there are two very distinct claims, each grounded in distributive justice, and that the two claims should give rise to two very different responses.

1. As a matter of fairness, women as individuals ought not to be excluded from research and its associated direct benefits.
2. As a matter of fairness, women as a class of persons ought not to be deprived of the benefits of research, generalizable knowledge, and the development of new therapies.

The first claim is related to a shift in public opinion about research. In the 1960s and 1970s the prevailing image of research was that it was a burden from which persons would want to be protected. Research was seen as dangerous and exploitative. In the 1980s, largely in response to the highly articulate and effective AIDS activists, research has come to be seen as beneficial. It is a context in which subjects can receive "promising new therapies" and medical care that is both excellent and free of charge. Hence, the argument that nobody should be deprived arbitrarily of access to such benefits.

A response to the first claim would be to open the doors to all persons, including women, to all research projects. The result would be the inclusion of varying numbers of men and women in studies. While this would satisfy the claims of equal access to putative benefits, it would not necessarily result in the development of either knowledge or products that were especially relevant to either men or women. At least theoretically, such an open door policy might make it much more difficult to develop knowledge or products especially relevant to either gender. For example, a drug that was more effective than placebo in women but not in men could, in a clinical trial involving both men and women, be found no better than placebo when the results obtained from both men and women were averaged together.

Now let us consider the second argument: that women as a class of persons ought not to be deprived of the benefits of research, generalizable knowledge, and the development of new therapies. A response to this claim does not entail establishing an open door policy. Rather, it involves the conduct of studies involving as subjects only men *and* only women *and,* in some cases, men and women in a design intended to compare them in a formal way. For example, one might develop a placebo-controlled, randomized clinical trial of a new drug in which an equal number of men and women would be enrolled and subjects would be stratified according to gender.

I think it is very important to be attentive to the differences in these two justice-based claims so that we can proceed intelligently to develop our research policies. The current National Institutes of Health policy calling for involvement of women and minorities in research unless their exclusion can be justified seems to be responsive only to the first of these two claims.

WOMEN IN (SOME) DEVELOPING COUNTRIES

Finally, I want to comment on a problem that we in the United States will find inescapable as it becomes necessary to conduct some studies involving subjects in developing countries. Time does not permit my providing an account of the intense arguments surrounding this issue. For the purpose of starting a discussion, I shall just read one paragraph from the recently published Council for International Organizations of Medical Sciences (CIOMS) *International*

Ethical Guidelines for Biomedical Research Involving Human Subjects (CIOMS, 1993):

> Obtaining the informed consent of women, including those who are pregnant or nursing, usually presents no special problems. In some cultures, however, women's rights to exercise self-determination and thus give valid informed consent are not acknowledged. In such cases, women should not normally be involved in research for which societies that recognize these rights require informed consent. Nevertheless, women who have serious illnesses or who are at risk of developing such illnesses should not be deprived of opportunities to receive investigational therapies when there are no better alternatives, even though they may not consent for themselves. Efforts must be made to let such women know of these opportunities and to invite them to decide whether they wish to accept the investigational therapy, even though the formal consent must be obtained from another person, usually a man. Such invitations may best be extended by women who understand the culture sufficiently well to discern whether prospective recipients of investigational therapies genuinely wish to accept or reject the therapy.

REFERENCES

Council for International Organizations of Medical Sciences in collaboration with the World Health Organization. 1993. International Ethical Guidelines for Biomedical Research Involving Human Subjects. Geneva: WHO.

Newton, L. 1984 Agreement to participate in research: Is that a promise? IRB: A Review of Human Subjects Research 6(2):7–99.

Impact of Current Federal Regulations on the Inclusion of Female Subjects in Clinical Studies

Vanessa Merton

THE IMPACT OF PRESENT LAW

Although clearly regulations that were adopted only 20 or so years ago cannot account for the longer history of exclusion of women from research, some researchers now say that they would be willing to include women in their protocols, were it not for the federal regulations that seem to them (or to their institutional review boards, or their institutions' lawyers) to prohibit or limit women's participation.[1] These regulations do indeed pose some obstacles and should be amended, but careful examination suggests that even in their present form, the federal regulations are by no means an insurmountable hurdle to the inclusion of women, including pregnant women, in biomedical protocols. Indeed, some federal regulations support and facilitate the participation of women in clinical research.

Regulations that Appear to Limit Women's Participation in Clinical Research

FDA Definition of "Childbearing Potential" and Required Prior Reproductive Studies

Research protocols commonly contain the exclusionary criterion "pregnant and lactating women and women of childbearing potential," language apparently derived from the Food and Drug Administration's Guidelines for researchers.[2] While the Guidelines are not legally binding, research conducted in accordance with the Guidelines qualifies for FDA consideration in a New Drug Application,[3] and most investigators take the Guidelines seriously. Certainly no prudent attorney would recommend their cavalier disregard, since they might well be deemed a "standard of care" for the research community.[4]

The Guidelines state that women of childbearing potential should be barred from large-scale (Phase III) clinical trials until all three segments of the FDA animal reproduction studies have been completed, and that women may be included in Phase II (controlled trials in several hundred subjects) studies only if "segment II and the female part of segment I of the FDA Animal Reproduction Guidelines have been completed."[5] Segment I covers gonadal function, effects of estrous cycles/mating behavior, and early gestation; segment II, teratogenesis; and segment III, the drug's effect on late fetal development, labor and delivery, lactation, and newborn health. (Remarkably, the Guidelines are silent on the question of how the *results* of the animal reproduction studies ought to affect inclusion or exclusion of women.)

There is no mandate to perform any of the animal reproduction studies *ever,* and certainly not prior to the conduct of Phase II or III trials.[6] The regulation that describes what applications for new drug approval must contain says only that the application should include nonclinical "studies, *as appropriate,* of the effects of the drug on reproduction and on the developing fetus."[7] Whether under this standard the FDA could approve a New Drug Application without animal testing for reproductive effect has never been determined by a court, so far as I can tell (probably because it would be extremely imprudent for a drug manufacturer not to do some such studies at some point prior to marketing),[8] but the FDA does not appear ever to have required such studies to precede Phase III trials.[9] There is no practical way for me to research this, but I would bet that "as appropriate" has never been interpreted to require animal studies that would elicit adverse reproductive effects mediated through the male animal.[10]

What this boils down to is that pharmaceutical companies can choose to market drugs with *no* information about their reproductive impact, so long as the label makes this clear,[11] and that the animal studies which the FDA defines as a necessary precursor to large-scale clinical trials with female subjects may never be conducted at all or may be done only in parallel with, not in advance of, clinical testing.

To compound this, the FDA, and thus clinical investigators, define the Guidelines' key phrase "of childbearing potential" in a way that, as I have written in another context, envisions all women as "constantly poised for reproductive activity":[12]

A woman of childbearing potential is defined as a premenopausal female capable of becoming pregnant. This includes women on oral, injectable, or mechanical contraception; women who are single; women whose husbands have been vasectomized or whose husbands have received or are utilizing mechanical contraceptive devices.[13]

The breadth of this definition of childbearing potential makes it tantamount to "all fertile women." The FDA limits the universe of women subjects right up through Phase III trials to "women who have been surgically sterilized, women who are postmenopausal, and women who are infertile . . . provided they [infertile women] are willing to use an effective form of contraception during the study, or have been evaluated by a fertility expert and have been found to be infertile, and have been so for greater than five years," to quote one research manual's interpretation.[14]

The FDA Guidelines do, however, expressly recognize an exception to the animal reproductive study requirement that gives researchers substantial latitude: testing of a drug anticipated to be a lifesaving or life-prolonging measure.[15] "Life-prolonging" seems a quite elastic phrase that could cover many situations of clinical research. Under the Guidelines, so long as the lack of reproduction studies is pointed out during the informed consent process, and she is tested for pregnancy and advised of contraceptive measures, the woman of childbearing potential may participate in clinical trials of a potentially life-prolonging intervention, even during Phase I. The nursing mother is specifically mentioned as a potential subject, with analysis of the excretion of the drug or its metabolites in the milk to be determined "when feasible."[16] And the one reference to pregnant women in the Guidelines merely notes that fetal follow-up should be carried out if a subject becomes pregnant while on the protocol;[17] it does not say anything about immediately terminating the woman from the protocol, a provision frequently found in research design.

The head of the FDA's Office on Drug Evaluation, Dr. Robert Temple, maintains that the Guidelines should not be interpreted by researchers to require the exclusion of women from protocols.[18] This observation is a welcome one, but apparently it has not been widely disseminated and is not widely shared by researchers.[19] The problem here may be largely one of misperception, which a vigorous effort by the agency could remedy.

DHHS Limitations on Research with Pregnant Women

The FDA Guidelines, then, can be parsed to have relatively little impact on women's participation in research, unless the researcher wants them to. The relevant Department of Health and Human Services (DHHS) regulations, on the other hand, appear to be a far greater constraint. However, they deal exclusively with the pregnant, rather than merely pregnable, woman.

Subpart B of Part 46 of Title 45 of the Code of Federal Regulations is entitled "Additional Protections Pertaining to Research, Development, and Related Activities Involving Fetuses, Pregnant Women, and Human In Vitro Fertilization." Promulgated in the mid-1970s, Subpart B prohibits research "involving" pregnant women unless (1) "appropriate" studies on animals and nonpregnant individuals have been completed;[20] (2) the purpose of the research is "to meet the health needs" of the woman; and (3) the fetus will be placed at minimal risk or at risk to the minimum extent necessary to meet the woman's health needs.[21]

So how significant a barrier for the pregnant woman are these regulations? To begin, let us consider the first requirement: completion of "appropriate" studies in animals and nonpregnant people (but presumably, under the Guidelines, not studies in women of childbearing potential). "Appropriate" is what lawyers call a weasel word, a word that gives the decision maker in a situation great discretion. Could this be a reference to teratogenicity studies? General clinical pharmacology studies for toxicity? Or perhaps the sort of *in vitro* work or uncontrolled case reports that one would ordinarily expect to foreshadow clinical research? It is hard to imagine the government's succeeding in imposing sanctions on a researcher for violating this amorphous provision unless absolutely no work had been done on the intervention on trial before the pregnant woman was permitted to participate.

More troubling is the requirement that the research be intended to "meet the health needs of the mother (sic)."[22] I will not try to improve on Robert Levine's trenchant exposition of the conceptual murkiness of the terms "therapeutic research" and "nontherapeutic research" and their especially problematic usage in this context.[23] Suffice it to say, this is another phrase that gives the researcher considerable scope. In a longer paper, I have identified the many ways in which participation in a research protocol in and of itself, regardless of the efficacy of the intervention on trial, may serve a subject's health needs.[24] I will add only that from the standpoint of psychic health, it takes a severe toll for a pregnant woman (or for any woman) to be told that after having been fully informed of the risks to her potential offspring, she cannot be trusted to decide whether to participate in a protocol, while no restrictions of any kind are placed on the decisions of her male counterpart, whose offspring may be at equal risk.

The final requirement is that the risk to the fetus must be minimal: again, an ill-defined and comparative term.[25] "Minimal risk" is defined elsewhere in the regulations to mean that the danger anticipated from the research is not greater, considering both probability and magnitude, than the danger of ordinary daily life or routine physical or psychological tests.[26] For a fetus, isn't an amniocentesis, with its half-percent chance of miscarriage, now a routine test? What about chorionic villi sampling? Ultrasound? Would the risk of ordinary daily life include the risk of a parent who smokes or who works where smoking is permitted? Drinks socially? Eats food containing additives? Disregards the prenatal care provider's advice?

But perhaps the more important question is, who should make this assessment? Is there reason to believe that the researcher, or perhaps the IRB, or perhaps a federal bureaucrat, is the best choice to judge the net of harm and benefit, risk and advantage, that would result from a pregnant woman's participation in a protocol?[27] Such a conclusion seems to presume maternal–fetal conflict, to ignore the inextricable link between the pregnant woman and the conceptus at any stage of its development, and to deny the woman's inherent responsibility for that part of her body which may be born a child.[28] As the DHHS regulations require, the woman must and should be fully informed about the risks, known and unknown, to her fetus. But nowhere do the regulations say, and no fair and rational reading can impute, that the judgment as to the requisite level of risk, and its proper weight in light of the woman's health needs, should be made by anyone other than her.[29] The absence of either administrative or judicial review of this question, as well as of the other questions raised by the DHHS regulations, underscores my conclusion that federal regulations are not trammeling researchers who in their eagerness to recruit and accept women subjects have been testing the boundaries of the law. The participation of women, and indeed of pregnant women, in clinical research is permitted, if complicated, by the federal regulations; the most problematic provisions probably would not survive scrutiny if challenged. But there have been no challenges, which seems to suggest that they are the product, not the cause, of the research tradition that excludes women for quite other reasons.

Federal Requirements that *Support* the Inclusion of Women in Clinical Research

FDA Premarketing Testing

Two different sources of law require adequate testing of pharmaceutical products. First, federal statutes and FDA regulations require that a New Drug Application demonstrate "adequate, and well-controlled investigations, including clinical investigations . . ."[30] and "data demonstrating substantial evidence of effectiveness for the claimed indications."[31] Second, it has long been recognized that the obligation to adequately test drugs before beginning to profit from their marketing is grounded in basic tort law principles. Beginning with the debacle of MER/29, the Richardson-Merrell anticholesterol product that blinded many people because the company failed to pursue ocular abnormalities in test animals,[32] courts have penalized companies that do not conduct reasonable testing to determine the potential adverse reactions of their products, even if the testing involved was not required by the FDA.[33]

In terms of the regulations, however, the question is, what do the phrases "adequate and well-controlled investigations" and "data demonstrating substantial effectiveness" mean? For the purposes of this discussion, one significant clue is the FDA's regulation on the labeling of drugs: "Evidence is . . . required to support the dosage and administration section of the labeling, and modifications for specific subgroups (for example, pediatrics, geriatrics, patients with renal failure)."[34] "If evidence is available to support the safety and effectiveness of the drug only in selected subgroups of the larger population . . . , the labeling shall describe the available evidence and state the limitations of the usefulness of the drug."[35]

Certainly it is reasonable to assert that with respect to the many interventions that have been tested only in male subjects, women are a "subgroup" for whom the data available is of limited utility. It is now uncontroversial that drug metabolism, dose-response reaction, and many other significant values, signs, and markers of clinical effect are different in women than in men.[36] A recent report of the Council on Ethical and Judicial Affairs of the American Medical Association documents numerous examples of disparities in providing women major diagnostic and therapeutic interventions, ranging from kidney dialysis and transplantation to diagnosis of lung cancer.[37] The Council concluded that these disparities could not be accounted for by biological differences or other benign or neutral variables. It found that "medical treatments for women are based on a male model, regardless of the fact that women may react differently to treatments than men or that some diseases manifest themselves differently in women than in men. The results of medical research on men are generalized to women without sufficient evidence of applicability to women."[38] The Council went on to recommend: "Research on health problems that affect both sexes should include male and female subjects. Sound medical and scientific reasons should be required for excluding women from medical tests and studies, such as that the proposed research does not or would not affect the health of women."[39]

Arguably, then, the FDA regulations should be read to require adequate testing, meaning sample sizes and/or stratified analyses sufficient to detect high-background adverse reactions, in a female population, unless the drug label reveals the paucity of data in women and cautions against undue extrapolation from testing in men.[40]

DHHS Regulations on Research with Children

One of the issues frequently raised in the course of discussing the enrollment of female subjects in clinical trials is the research sponsor's concern about liability to their offspring.[41] In that context, it is sometimes said that this concern cannot be resolved by any sort of "waiver" or "assumption of risk" by parent-subjects on behalf of their offspring, because while parents can consent to their children's participation in all manner of fairly dangerous and nonbeneficial activities outside the medical arena, generally they can consent to medical intervention for their children only if the intervention is intended and expected to be beneficial to the individual child.[42] The traditional view, therefore, has been that parents lack capacity to consent to their child's participation in nontherapeutic research, and therefore, *ipso facto,* to assumption of the risks of the child's participation in such research, although the one attempt to obtain a judicial declaration that parents have no right either to permit or to compel their children's participation in nontherapeutic research did not succeed.[43]

The analogy between parental assumption of risk for born, living children who are *themselves* the subjects of research, and release of a sponsor from responsibility for harm to a subject's unborn or unconceived children, is tenuous at best, but federal regulations become relevant here because of their explicit recognition that parents can consent to nontherapeutic research (and therefore, logically, to assumption of the risks of that research). In 1983 the DHHS promulgated regulations that clearly contemplate and authorize parental consent to a broad range of nontherapeutic research with child subjects.[44] It is hard to imagine that the lengthy provisions of these regulations which describe in detail the quality of consent necessary for such research[45] will be treated as nugatory in any future liability litigation, rather than as the source of public policy they obviously are.

RECOMMENDED CHANGES IN THE FEDERAL LAW

Full inclusion of women in biomedical research would be somewhat easier to implement if there were some revision of current federal regulations. Because these limitations are not statutory in origin, however, such revision would not require congressional action, but could be undertaken by the relevant administrative agencies at any time.[46]

Amendment of FDA Regulations

First, the FDA Guidelines should be redrafted to raise identical concerns about the participation of both male and female subjects of reproductive potential, and to allow women to decide for themselves, as men do, about the relative risks and benefits—for them—of participation in Phase I or early Phase II trials.[47] FDA regulations require researchers to inform subjects "when appropriate" that the research may involve "risks to the subject (or to the embryo or fetus, if the subject is or may become pregnant) which are currently unforeseeable."[48] This section should be amended to require researchers also to inform male subjects who are or may become involved in reproductive activity of the state of knowledge about male-transmitted birth defects and/or effects on male germ cells.[49] In many cases the current knowledge will be nil; nothing will be known because the intervention has not been tested on this parameter.

Subjects should be told this, and told also that while instances of adverse reproductive effect for or through the male parent have occurred, too little is yet known to permit quantification of the risk. If women are required to use contraception, then so should men.[50]

The most efficient method of changing researcher behavior would be to amend the substantive provisions of FDA regulations to require complete testing of new drugs in relevant populations, specifically women of childbearing age, pregnant women, and nursing women.[51] At a minimum, the FDA ought to ensure that drug labels state that evidence of both safety and efficacy is lacking for these populations whenever that is the case, and that nothing is known about reproductive hazards for men, which will almost invariably be the case.

Amendment of DHHS Regulations

The only major change needed in the Federal Policy for the Protection of Human Subjects is in the section on equitable selection of subjects, Section III. "Pregnant women" should either be removed from the category of "vulnerable populations" or replaced by "men and women actively engaged in reproduction." To amplify the definition of "equitable," helpful language may be borrowed from a fine consensus document by a working group on principles and policies for clinical research on HIV infection, which concluded that:

> No group should be categorically excluded, on the basis of age, gender, mental status, place of residence or incarceration, or other social or economic characteristic from access to clinical trials or other mechanisms of access to experimental therapies. Special efforts should be made to reach out to previously excluded populations. . . . It is inequitable and discriminatory to exclude women, including women of reproductive age, from clinical trials.[52]

Another component of DHHS regulations that needs revision is Subpart B. Here, the best option would be to delete Section 46.207, the provision dealing with "Activities directed toward pregnant women as subjects." Its language is ambiguous and confusing; the subsection requiring paternal consent is surely unconstitutional even under present standards; and given that about all it permits is activity intended to "meet the health needs of the mother," depending on one's view of the purposes of clinical research, either it is tautological or it describes a null set. The bulk of the other provisions of Subpart B, which govern fetal research, suffer from various infirmities and illogicalities that ought to be corrected, but do not in themselves pose any particular barrier to women's participation in protocols.

National Institutes of Health Policy

The National Institutes of Health can itself, through implementation of its own policy,[53] dramatically influence the pattern of excluding women from biomedical research. But to do so, more specific standards than are contained in the current policy are necessary. The NIH/ADAMHA Policy Concerning Inclusion of Women in Study Populations ("NIH Policy") appears to establish a firm presumption that women *shall* be included in protocols. However, that presumption may be rebutted by showing either (1) that it would be "inappropriate" to include women in a given study; or (2) a "compelling justification" for the exclusion of women. In conjunction, these criteria for exemption from the policy are quite capable of swallowing it whole—the proverbial Mack truck would have no trouble navigating these holes.

For example, the NIH Policy states that "appropriateness" of inclusion of women is in part a function of the "known incidence/prevalence" of a condition among women. Yet one of the major consequences of the exclusion of women from research has been enormous gaps in existing knowledge about the epidemiology of many conditions in women. As the members of the Women in Research Task Force, a bioethics group in which I participated, wrote in a letter to Dr. Kirschstein, then Acting Associate Director of the new NIH Office of Research on Women's Health, "Thus, women could end up being excluded from a study based on data from studies which excluded women in the first place."[54] Moreover, women must be leery of terms like "appropriate" when those who will be deciding what they mean remain overwhelmingly products of the mind set and world view that has so often found subordination, denigration, and paternalistic protection of women "appropriate."

Likewise, with respect to the "compelling justification" for exclusion of women, to exempt a protocol from the NIH Policy, researchers may need only recite the usual claims about "dirty data" or fear of liability. In its Memorandum OER 90-5, NIH refers to two situations that qualify as "compelling": (1) the condition to be studied occurs only in men; or (2) inclusion of women would "jeopardize the health and safety" of a class of subjects. Without clarification, it is not hard to imagine that fetal protection may be the hidden meaning of the latter. I find disquieting, rather than comforting, Dr. Kirschstein's response to the Women in Research Task Force letter, in which she states:

A list of situations that comprehensively accounts for all such justifications for "compelling" exclusion is very difficult to create. . . . One potential basis . . . is the case in which the financial and human costs of conducting research trials are significantly increased or unduly burdensome in comparison to the benefit gained by including a representative number of both genders in the study population for a disease or condition in which the incidence is lower in one gender than in the other. . . . Another potential basis for rebuttal is the situation in which violation of the established legal rights of a child or potential rights of a fetus are a foreseeable possibility as a result of the mother's participation in a clinical trial. ... [C]ases in which studies on animals measuring teratogenic or other significant adverse effects are incomplete or inconclusive warrant exclusion justification review and may serve as sufficient grounds for rebutting the inclusion presumption.[55]

Several questions are raised by this response. First, when Dr. Kirschstein speaks of "financial and human costs of conducting research trials," I wonder whose costs, or costs to whom? For women as a class, the cost of their involuntary nonparticipation in research has long outweighed the benefit. Second, what "potential rights of a fetus" (or, for that matter, established rights of a child) are violated when a woman chooses to take an unapproved drug? Surely those same rights, whatever they may be, are violated when the same woman now takes an approved drug that has never been tested in women, or in pregnant women, but is available on the market, or when the woman fails to follow a doctor's orders, or to exercise regularly, or to do a thousand other things that are "good" for her—as, once upon a time, thalidomide, diethylstilbestrol, diuretics, X-rays, routine cesarean section, and minimal weight gain were deemed "good" for pregnant women by their physicians. With this language, I am afraid Dr. Kirschstein and the Office of Research on Women's Health, the putative bastion of women's rights and liberties in this process, inadvertently reinforce the coercive, intrusive model of "maternal–fetal (or child) conflict."[56]

As for "incomplete or inconclusive" animal studies of teratogenicity or "other significant adverse effects [presumably, upon reproductive outcomes]," so far as I am aware, there is nothing but incomplete, inconclusive data in this area; for a start, the absence of such studies with respect to male-mediated effects on offspring render them all, by definition, partial and inconclusive. If Dr. Kirschstein's statement is taken literally, hardly any research should be permitted.

There is an alternative approach: requiring adequate animal studies of adverse reproductive effects in both male and female animals. Such studies would have to test for all potential male routes of prenatal and preconceptual impact. If NIH is serious about avoiding risk to the offspring of research subjects, the only effective method is either to permit participation only of nonfertile men and women—difficult for large-scale studies, and unlikely to be clinically representative—or to impose much more rigorous controls on reproductive behavior by human study participants, both male and female.[57]

CONCLUSION

There is much more, beyond fixing specific regulations, that all the federal agencies—NIH, DHHS, and FDA—could do to redress the current situation. Gender-specific and gender-comparative research that will provide better understanding of the etiology and risk factors for disease in women ought to receive priority in funding and other resources. Federal agencies should require that *all* research be evaluated to determine whether its design will elucidate gender-specific differences and permit systematic analyses of gender-specific variables.[58] This requirement cannot be confined to areas of acknowledged gender difference, for example, drugs metabolized through pathways influenced by sex steroid hormones, because the failure to recognize differences may reflect a lack of prior research rather than the right questions having been asked and answered in the negative.[59] At a minimum, pharmacokinetic screens of all new drugs should be conducted in both women and men, and animal studies should include female as well as male animals. Whenever animal reproductive studies are conducted, they should seek to determine the incidence of adverse reproductive outcomes through the male parent.

In the eloquent words of the executive director of the Center for Women Policy Studies, "research must study women in their own right, and on their own biological terms, not as if they were defective men."[60] Especially when research is conducted with government funds, subject to government control, in government facilities by government-supported or government-trained researchers, there can be no justification for validating the safety and efficacy of an intervention only in men. Nothing less than the health of our daughters is at stake.

NOTES

1. I should note that these regulations technically apply only to certain classes of clinical research, albeit the central ones. The Food and Drug Administration (FDA) regulations govern research intended to obtain approval for commercial distribution of a new drug or device (or of an approved drug/device for a new indication). In June 1991 the "Basic HHS Policy for Protection of Human Research Subjects" (also known as "Subpart A") was replaced by a new Federal Policy for the Protection of Human Subjects. *See* 45 C.F.R. Part 46 (1992); Joan Porter, "The Federal Policy for the Protection of Human Subjects," *IRB: A Review of Human Subjects Research* 13: 8–9, at 8 (September–October 1991). This new policy, adopted as a common rule by 16 federal agencies and departments, applies not only to research funded by, but subject to regulation from, any of these agencies and departments. However, Subpart B, Department of Health and Human Services (DHHS) regulations pertinent to research with pregnant women, applies only to research conducted or supported in whole or in part with HHS funds. As a practical matter, however, most privately funded institutions and researchers operate according to these rules.

2. Food and Drug Administration, *General Considerations for the Clinical Evaluation of Drugs.* Washington, D.C.: U.S. Government Printing Office, FDA Publication 77-3040 (1977) [hereinafter, Guidelines].

On the morning of March 25, 1993, approximately 10 minutes before the presentation of this paper at the Institute of Medicine Workshop, Dr. Ruth Merkatz, Special Assistant on Women's Health to the Commissioner of the Food and Drug Administration, announced that the FDA was substantially amending the *Guidelines* to eliminate the ban on participation of fertile women in early trials and to require analysis of data to detect gender differences in the activity or effects of a drug. As of this writing, the actual text of the new policy had not been released to the public, so it was impossible to assess its impact. Dr. David A. Kessler, FDA Commissioner, has been quoted as saying that the agency "reserves the right not to approve their [New Drug Applications]" in reference to researchers who did not include "enough women." Philip J. Hilts, "F.D.A. Ends Ban on Women in Drug Testing," *New York Times*, March 25, 1993, p. B8, col. 4. However, based on the responses of Dr. Merkatz to questions at the workshop, it appears that the new rule does not *mandate* the participation of a proportionate number of women in protocols, but merely removes the language, discussed herein, that has frequently been cited as the basis for their exclusion. It still requires only women, not men, to abstain from reproductive behavior while on protocol, and continues to dictate exclusion of pregnant and lactating women. The new policy also does not compel research sponsors to complete animal reproduction studies in both male and female animals prior to commencement of clinical trials. My own expectation is that absent regulatory compulsion, liability concerns and some of the other factors discussed at the workshop will remain formidable obstacles to the participation of women as subjects in biomedical research.

3. 21 C.F.R. § 10.90(b) (1992) (research conducted in good faith pursuant to Guidelines will be accepted by FDA for review). "A person may rely upon a guideline with assurance that it is acceptable to FDA. . . ." *Id.* at § 10.90(b)(1)(i).

4. Knowing its visceral impact, I prefer to avoid using the word "malpractice" in a paper intended for health professionals, but I should explain this reference for those unfamiliar with the phrase "standard of care": a patient or a client in a professional relationship who seeks to hold the professional responsible for a bad outcome must prove, among other things, that the harm would not have occurred had the professional not breached a professional standard of care; that is, did not provide care within the broad range of choices that a competent professional might reasonably consider under the circumstances. Protocols and standards issued by professional organizations and governmental agencies sometimes are utilized as sources of the "standard of care." *See* Steven E. Pegalis and Harvey F. Wachsman, *American Law of Medical Malpractice 2d* §§ 3.1–3.13, 85–176. Deerfield, IL: Clark Boardman Callaghan (1992). Specifically, the FDA's own regulations provide that "[a] guideline may be used in administrative or court proceedings to illustrate acceptable and unacceptable procedures or standards." 21 C.F.R. § 10.90(b)(8) (1992).

5. Guidelines at 10. For a good description of the Phase I-Phase II-Phase III categories by the Commissioner of the Food and Drug Administration, *see* David Kessler, "The Regulation of Investigational Drugs," *New England Journal of Medicine* 320: 218–288, 282 (February 2, 1989).

6. Some texts and treatises seem to assume that this testing is necessary for a New Drug Application. *See* Donald E. Vinson and Alexander H. Slaughter, *Products Liability: Pharmaceutical Drug Cases* § 5.04 at 210. Colorado Springs, CO: Shepard's/ McGraw-Hill (1988 and 1991 Suppl.). But nothing in the language of the regulations or the *Guidelines* is couched in mandatory rather than precatory terms.

7. 21 C.F.R. § 314.50(d)(2)(iii) (1992) (emphasis added).

8. In a much longer paper on this subject I describe the common-law duty of drug manufacturers to conduct adequate product testing, which is quite distinct from requirements imposed by the FDA. *See* Vanessa Merton, "The Exclusion of Pregnant, Pregnable, and Once-Pregnable People (a.k.a. Women) From Biomedical Research" (1992) (manuscript on file with the author, to be published in late 1993 in *The American Journal of Law and Medicine)* [hereinafter Merton, "The Exclusion of Pregnant, Pregnable, and Once-Pregnable People"].

9. Dr. Robert Temple, Director of the Office on Drug Evaluation of the Food and Drug Administration, has stated that no one at the FDA is responsible for determining whether animal reproduction studies are actually conducted. Response to question at Institute of Medicine workshop on women and drug development, June 23, 1992.

10. The Guidelines do suggest that when testicular or spermatogenetic abnormalities have been observed in animals (which is not to say that animal studies to evoke these responses must be done), or when chromosomal abnormalities are anticipated, the inclusion of males in all three phases of trials depends on a constellation of factors: the nature of the abnormalities, the "importance" of the drug, etc. Compare this textured, case-by-case, only-if-reason-for-concern-has-been-demonstrated approach to the categorical language of the rule about women of childbearing potential, *infra* at p. 3. There is also no mention of a need to discuss contraception with male subjects in these circumstances.

11. 21 C.F.R. § 201.57 (1992), which governs labeling of human prescription drugs, requires a statement of critical information, *if known*, but does not create any independent duty to acquire the information. For example, under subsections (f)(5) and (6), the label must specify whether "adequate and well-controlled studies in pregnant women" have or have not demonstrated a risk to the fetus, and describe the results of animal reproduction studies, *if* available. But it is perfectly acceptable to label a drug Pregnancy Category C, in the event that there are no animal reproduction studies and no studies in humans, and state that "It is also not known whether *(name of drug)* can cause fetal harm when administered to a pregnant woman or can affect reproduction capacity. *(Name of drug)* should be given to a pregnant woman only if clearly needed." Even under the category of nonteratogenic effects, in subsection (f)(6)(ii), there is no requirement to provide either information, or a warning of the absence of information, about the drug's reproductive impact in men.

12. Vanessa Merton, "Community-Based AIDS Research," *Evaluation Review* 14: 502–537, 519 (October 1990).

13. *Guidelines* at 10.

14. Frank L. Iber, W. Anthony Riley, and Patricia J. Murray, *Conducting Clinical Trials* 179. New York and London: Plenum Medical Book Company (1987).

15. *Guidelines* at 10.

16. *Id.* at 11.

17. *Id.*

18. Interview with Robert Temple and Margaret Jensvold, *FDA Consumer* 25: 8 (April 1991); *see also* Carol Levine, "Women and HIV/AIDS Research," *Evaluation Review* 14:447–463, 455 (October 1990).

19. In a confidential 1991 survey conducted by the Pharmaceutical Manufacturers Association, 79 percent of the 33 companies surveyed reported that FDA reviewers had required them to exclude women of childbearing potential from their protocols. Lionel D. Edwards, "Design and Conduct of Research in Women: To Include or Exclude: A Pharmaceutical Industry Physician's Perspective" (1992)(unpublished manuscript on file with the author) [hereinafter, Edwards, "Design and Conduct of Research"].

20. 45 C.F.R. § 46.206 (1992). Other conditions, intended to ensure that no inducements or pressures to terminate the pregnancy are part of the research design, are also enumerated in this section.

21. 45 C.F.R. § 46.207 (1992). Section 46.205 imposes various special obligations, mostly pertaining to informed consent, on IRBs that review protocols involving pregnant women and fetuses. All these provisions may be waived or modified by the Secretary of Health and Human Services on request of a researcher, 45 C.F.R. § 46.211 (1992), but virtually no requests have been made, possibly because since 1980 an indispensable participant in the waiver process, an Ethical Advisory Board within HHS, has not been funded or appointed. *See* Robert Levine, *Ethics and Regulation of Clinical Research* 319–320, New Haven and London: Yale University Press (2d ed. 1988) [hereinafter, Levine, *Ethics and Regulation*].

22. A pregnant woman is not yet a mother, and her impregnator is not yet a father. *See* Renee Solomon, "Future Fear: Prenatal Duties Imposed by Private Parties," *American Journal of Law and Medicine* 17:411,434,417, n. 37 (1991).

23. Levine, *Ethics and Regulation*, 8–10, 298.

24. *See* Merton, "The Exclusion of Pregnant, Pregnable, and Once-Pregnable People."

25. *See* Joseph F. Fletcher and Joseph D. Schulman, "Fetal Research: The State of the Question," *Hastings Center Report* 15:6–12 (April 1985), and Karen Lebacqz, "Fetal Research; A Commissioner's Reflection," *IRB: A Review of Human Subjects Research* 1:7–8 (June/July 1979), for varied approaches to assessing risk in this context.

26. 45 C.F.R. § 46.102(i) (1992).

27. A further provision tries to require that the "father" of the fetus (to use the loaded language of the section, *see* n. 22 supra) give his informed consent to the pregnant woman's participation in the research. Presumably unintentionally, however, the drafters rendered this provision meaningless. The various exceptions to the progenitor-consent requirement are stated in the disjunctive, that is, any one of them permits departure from the rule. One exception is identical to a precondition for the pregnant woman's participation in research that may pose more than a minimal risk to the fetus: i.e., that the purpose of the research be to meet the pregnant woman's health needs. Since any research that poses more than minimal risk is permissible *only* if its purpose is to meet the pregnant woman's health needs (regardless of progenitor consent), this exception will almost always subsume the apparent requirement of progenitor consent. Progenitor consent is actually necessary only when (1) the risk to the fetus is minimal (or less); and (2) the research can in no way be characterized as directed toward the woman's health

needs. Other exceptions to this requirement also might be applicable to many pregnant research subjects: when the father cannot be identified or found, or the pregnancy results from rape.

Given the recent Supreme Court decision in *Planned Parenthood of Southeastern Pennsylvania v. Casey*, 112 S.Ct. 2791 (1992), it is hard to see how this paternal consent condition, if ever applied, would survive constitutional challenge. The only antichoice state restriction struck down by *Casey* was the husband notification provision, because "it cannot be claimed that the father's interest in the fetus' welfare is equal to the mother's protected liberty, since it is an inescapable biological fact that state regulation with respect to the fetus will have a far greater impact on the pregnant woman's bodily integrity than it will on the husband." 112 S.Ct. 2799–2800. If paternal *notification* cannot be required for an abortion, the constitutionality of requiring paternal *consent* for a much lesser risk to the fetus is dubious.

28. The subject of "maternal–fetal conflict," and the fallacious and invidious premises packed into that term, are ably dissected in Dawn Johnsen, "Shared Interests: Promoting Healthy Births without Sacrificing Women's Liberty," *Hastings Law Journal* 43:569–614 (1992).

29. *See* National Commission for the Protection of Human Subjects of Biomedical and Behavioral Research, *Research on the Fetus*. Washington, D.C.: U.S. Government Printing Office, DHEW Publication No. (OS) 76-127 (1975) at 65:

Therapeutic research directed toward the pregnant woman may expose the fetus to risk for the benefit of another subject and thus is at first glance more problematic. Recognizing the woman's priority regarding her own health care, however, the Commission concludes that such research is ethically acceptable provided that the woman has been fully informed of the possible impact on the fetus and that other general requirements have been met. Protection for the fetus is further provided by requiring that research put the fetus at minimum risk consistent with the provision of health care for the woman. Moreover, therapeutic research directed toward the pregnant woman frequently benefits the fetus, though it need not necessarily do so. In view of the woman's right to privacy regarding her own health care, the Commission concludes that the informed consent of the woman is both necessary and sufficient.

In general, the Commission concludes that therapeutic research directed toward the health condition of either the fetus or the pregnant woman is, in principle, ethical. Such research benefits not only the individual woman or fetus but also women and fetuses as a class, and should therefore be encouraged actively.

30. 21 U.S.C. § 355 (1972 and 1992 Suppl.).

31. 21 C.F.R. § 314.50(d)(5)(v) (1992).

32. *Toole v. Richardson-Merrell, Inc.*, 60 Cal. Rptr. 398 (Dist. Ct. App. 1967).

33. *Barson v. E.R. Squibb & Sons, Inc.*, 682 P.2d 832 (Utah 1984) (manu-facturer negligent in not testing for teratogenic effects of injected progestational hormone).

34. 21 C.F.R. § 314.50(d)(5)(v) (1992).

35. 21 C.F.R. SS 201.57(c)(3)(i) (1992).

36. *See, e.g.,* Allen Raskin, "Age-Sex Differences in Response to Anti-depressant Drugs," *Journal of Nervous and Mental Diseases* 159:120–130 (1974) and many other references in Edwards, "Design and Conduct of Research in Women." Despite the extensive references he cites, demonstrating substantial gender differences in absorption kinetics and metabolism of such major drugs as propranolol, diazepam, and lithium, Dr. Edwards believes that the detectable differences are usually not therapeutically significant. His only authority for this proposition is his own previous work. *Id.* at 4, n. 13.

37. Council Report, "Gender Disparities in Clinical Decision Making," *Journal of the American Medical Association* 266:559–562 (July 24/31, 1991).

38. *Id.* at 559.

39. *Id.* at 562.

40. Although this goes beyond the scope of my report, a similar obligation to test in populations that reflect the population in which the manufacturer wants to market may be derived from the law of products liability. *See West v. Johnson & Johnson Products, Inc.,* 174 Cal.App.3d 831, 220 Cal. Rptr. 437, 448, 59 A.L.R. 4th 1, CCH Prod. Liab. Rep. 1 Para. 10,883 (1985) (plaintiff compensated because of failure of tampon manufacturer to study the basic microbiology of the human vagina, to test for vaginal infections, and—of particular interest—to include women with a history of vaginitis in clinical studies); *Taylor v. Wyeth Laboratories,* 362 N.W.2d 293, 296-97 (Mich. App. 1984) (even absent any study, prudent manufacturer would have explored relationship between blood type and blood-clotting risk in women taking oral contraceptives, once aware that women with type A blood experience disproportionate number of pulmonary embolisms). "Testing procedures should simulate as closely as possible the anticipated conditions of marketing and use of the product." Marden G. Dixon and Frank C. Woodside III, *Drug Product Liability* § 14.04 [2] at 14–68, New York: Matthew Bender (1990).

41. This subject is addressed in the companion paper of Professor Ellen Wright Clayton, "Liability Exposure When Offspring Are Injured as a Result of Parent Participation in Clinical Trials." In my own analysis of the question elsewhere, I have emphasized that researchers have as much cause for concern about liability to the offspring of their male subjects. *See* Merton, "The Exclusion of Pregnant, Pregnable, and Once-Pregnable People."

42. See *generally,* James M. Morrissey, Adele A. Hofmann, and Jeffrey C. Thrope, *Consent and Confidentiality in the Health Care of Children and Adolescents: A Legal Guide* 22, 90–91, New York: Free Press (1986). One *sui generis* situation that severely strains this precept is the case of a child who needs a bone marrow or kidney transplant that could best be supplied by a minor (or mentally impaired adult) sibling. May the parent consent to the healthy sibling's organ donation? Courts have permitted such procedures on theories of psychological benefit to the sibling or under the rubric of "substituted judgment"—the legal fiction that the child, if able to exercise judgment, would consent to the donation. *See Strunk v. Strunk,* 445 S.W.2d 145 (Ky. 1969); *Hart v. Brown,* 289 A.2d 386 (Conn. 1972). Other courts, however, have refused to honor the parents' wishes. *See,* e.g., *In re Richardson,* 284 So.2d 185 (La. 1973).

43. *Nielson v. Regents of University of California*, No. 660-047 (Sup. Ct. Cal. 1973) (unpublished disposition).

44. Subpart D: Additional Protections for Children Involved as Subjects in Research, 45 C.F.R. §§ 46.401 *et seq.* (1992). Permitted studies include research that presents "an opportunity to understand, prevent, or alleviate a serious problem affecting the health or welfare of children," 45 C.F.R. §§ 46.407 (1992), and research that presents greater than minimal risk and no prospect of direct benefit to the subject, but that is likely to yield "generalizable knowledge about the subject's . . . condition that is of vital importance for the understanding or amelioration of [that condition]." 45 C.F.R. §§ 46.406 (1992).

45. Instead of the term "consent," the regulations speak of parental *permission* and the child-subject's *assent*. IRBs may waive the requirement of parental permission and/or minor assent altogether. 45 C.F.R. § 46.408 (1992).

46. Legislatures enact statutes that define broad mandates for governmental agencies: to clean up the environment, protect worker health and safety, promote development of nuclear energy, etc. The individual agencies then adopt myriad detailed regulations through a process that may receive legislative scrutiny but does not require legislative approval. A regulation may be challenged in court as invalid because it is contrary to the express language or the purpose of the "enabling" statute, but in that event, the agency's own interpretation of the statute as embodied in the regulation will be given due deference by the reviewing court. *See generally, Chevron U.S.A. Inc. v. Natural Resources Defense Council, Inc., et al.*, 467 U.S. 837, 842–845 (1983).

47. As noted supra at n. 2, the proposed amendment of the Guidelines announced on March 24, 1993, does not address many of the concerns raised in the following discussion.

48. 21 C.F.R. § 50.25(b)(1) (1992).

49. In December 1992 a coalition of the HIV Law Project of the AIDS Service Center of Lower Manhattan, the National Organization for Women Legal Defense and Education Fund, the AIDS Project of the American Civil Liberties Union, and other AIDS-activist organizations petitioned the FDA for just such amendments, pursuant to 21 C.F.R. § 10.30 (1992). *See* Citizen Petition, copy on file with the author.

50. See infra n. 57 on the need for careful monitoring of male compliance with such restrictions.

51. A concomitant of this change would be for FDA regulations to mandate completion of animal reproduction studies prior to human testing. *See* Citizen Petition, supra n. 49.

52. Carol Levine, Nancy Neveloff Dubler, and Robert J. Levine, "Building a New Consensus: Ethical Principles and Policies for Clinical Research on HIV/AIDS," *IRB: A Review of Human Subjects Research* 13: 1–17, 14 and 16 (January–April 1991). The working group that developed this consensus document included prominent clinical AIDS researchers and ethicists, as well as representatives of potential subject populations. Their recommendations depart from mine in continuing to treat pregnant women as different from men engaged in reproductive activity, although they do require that pregnant women be permitted access to Phase II/III trials or treatment INDs if a drug is potentially lifesaving, and would create a rebuttable presumption that pregnant women are eligible for all trials. *See* id. at 16. While the context of this report is AIDS research, the merit

of its analysis is not confined to that.

53. In 1986, the National Institutes of Health (NIH) and the Alcohol, Drug Abuse, and Mental Health Administration (ADAMHA) promulgated the "Policy Concerning Inclusion of Women in Study Populations" (NIH Guide, Vol. 20, No. 6, February 8, 1991, pp. 1–2). "Clinical research findings should be of benefit to all persons at risk of the disease, regardless of gender." The policy requires evaluation of the gender composition of each study proposed for funding, and a statement of reasons for excluding members of one gender or for "a disproportionate representation" of one gender. Gender representation should be "appropriate to the known incidence/prevalence of the disease or condition being studied," and reasons for exclusion of one gender must be "well-explained and justified." The justification must be "compelling," but it may consist of "a strong scientific rationale" or "a need to protect the health of the subjects."

On its face, the policy sounds very promising. Unfortunately, it went unenforced and essentially disregarded for the first five years of its existence, as was documented in widely publicized congressional hearings and a Government Accounting Office report. The policy was not even published in the application booklet. Reviewers were instructed not to consider the inclusion of women as a factor of scientific merit. No one was denied funding for lack of gender representativeness; no records were kept about the demographics of protocols submitted and funded; and the policy applied only to extramural research, not intramural programs. *See* Mark V. Nadel, "National Institutes of Health: Problems in Implementing Policy on Women in Study Populations," Testimony before the Subcommittee on Health and the Environment, House of Representatives, June 18, 1990.

54. Letter of the Women in Research Task Force to Ruth L. Kirschstein, M.D., June 28, 1991 (on file with the author), p. 2.

55. Letter to Karen L. Hagberg, Coordinator, Women in Research Task Force, from Dr. Kirschstein, October 23, 1991 (on file with the author), p. 3.

56. *See* n. 28 supra.

57. Since it is more difficult to monitor male compliance with protocol restrictions on impregnation than to require routine pregnancy tests, more stringent limitations on the mobility, privacy, etc., of male subjects may be necessary for the duration of their study participation, and substantially thereafter, until it is established that their sperm are free of any contamination or mutation.

58. One of the very best sources of guidance on specific biostatistical analyses that ought to be performed, and other ideas for gender-neutral research design, remains Jean Hamilton, "Avoiding Methodological and Policy-Making Biases in Gender-Related Health Research," in *Women's Health: Report of the Public Health Service Task Force on Women's Health Issues IV*-54 to IV-64, IV-57 to IV-60. Washington, D.C.: U.S. Department of Health and Human Services, DHHS Publication No. (PHS) 88-50206 (1987). It is not yet clear whether the FDA's proposed new policy, *see* supra n. 2, actually requires proper research design, or merely that a stratification analysis of male and female subjects be performed, regardless of the persuasiveness of the results (e.g., even if the female sample size is inadequate).

59. *See* Institute of Medicine, *Expanding Access to Investigational Therapies for HIV Infection and AIDS* 7. Washington, D.C.: National Academy Press (1991).

60. Statement of Dr. Leslie Wolfe, submitted to the Task Force on Opportunities for Research on Women's Health, June 3, 1991 (on file with the author), at p. 8.

Brief Overview of Constitutional Issues Raised by the Exclusion of Women from Research Trials

R. Alta Charo

The exclusion of fertile women from research trials, based upon both FDA regulation and the pattern of practice among private pharmaceutical companies and academic centers, is *prima facie* disparate treatment of two classes of persons: fertile females and all others. Whether the disparate treatment of these two classes raises constitutional issues depends upon a number of factors:

1. Does the disparate treatment result in any disparate benefits to the two classes?
2. If so, are these benefits classified as specially protected "rights"?
3. Whether or not the benefits are classified as "rights," is there a justification for the disparate treatment, in light of the disparate benefits?
4. If so, does the disparity in benefit operate to disadvantage a protected class of persons? If it does, the level of justification for the disparate treatment must be somewhat higher.

This author concludes that the exclusion of fertile women does have the effect of denying women as a class an equal opportunity to benefit from government-funded research. The justifications for the exclusion, which rest primarily upon calls to protect potential fetuses from harm or to minimize the costs of research, are only dubiously sufficient to sustain the exclusion. Exclusion of women from nongovernmentally funded research, however, is probably constitutional.

DISPARATE TREATMENT, DISPARATE BENEFITS, AND EQUAL OPPORTUNITY

1. Does disparate treatment result in any disparate benefits to the two classes?

The goal of excluding fertile women from research trials is often achieved by excluding all women or all pre-menopausal women from the trial (Nadel, M.V., "NIH: Problems in Implementing Policy on Women in Study Populations," GAO/Y-HRD-90-38). Even where sterile women are included, many are sterile owing to hysterectomy, thus rendering their hormonal patterns unrepresentative of the hormonal patterns in fertile women (Cotton, 1990). The degree to which the operation of various drugs and therapeutic protocols differs in women and men, or fertile women and all others, is unclear. Inadequate data exists, whether at *in vitro*, animal, or human levels, to accurately predict which interventions are likely to be significantly affected by the different average body weight, body composition, hormonal patterns, and collateral diseases or drugs used by men and women (Cotton, 1990).

Nonetheless, tantalizing data do suggest that these differences exist more often than had been suspected. This paper, which focuses on constitutional issues, will not review those data. (But see GAO, "Women's Health: FDA Needs to Ensure More Study of Gender Difference in Prescription Drug Testing," GAO/HRD-93-17, October 1992; SAWHR, 1991). Instead, it is written on the assumption that further research would reveal that many, but not all, drugs and therapeutic interventions have different degrees of risk and efficacy in male and female populations.

2. Are the benefits of being a research subject specially protected "rights"?

Robert Levine has amply demonstrated that there has been a paradigm shift in the way in which we view enrollment in research trials (Levine, 1988). While research on human subjects was first viewed as a necessary aspect of public health, and then viewed as a transgression of individual rights tantamount to torture, it has lately come to be viewed as an avenue of access to better medical care for oneself and one's cohort, 1991.

Thus, being a research subject is no longer viewed as an unqualified sacrifice. Rather, it is a potentially risky opportunity. The degree of risk depends upon the nature of the therapy being tested and the fragility of the subject. The degree of opportunity depends upon the extent to which the subject suffers from a disorder destined to be treated by the therapy, the availability of effective therapeutic interventions already on the market, the urgency of the subject's disorder, and the access the subject has to paid, therapeutic care.

Looked at this way, fertile women who are denied access to clinical trials may or may companies ornot be denied a benefit. The question of benefit is idiosyncratic. To the extent, however, that the exclusion of fertile women from research trials does bar access for some to potentially lifesaving treatments (IOM, "Expanding Access to Investigational Therapies for HIV Infection and AIDS," 1991), it is undoubtedly the denial of a benefit. Further, if the exclusion of fertile women results in all women, as a class, being denied adequate protection from the marketing of drugs and interventions dangerous to their health, then this exclusion denies all women an important benefit of research. In other words, by failing to adequately test drugs and interventions on women during the premarketing phase of development, the female consumers of those products in the postmarketing phase are transformed into unwitting subjects of a poorly controlled and poorly monitored large-scale, long-term research trial.

Although there is no "right" to health care or to the benefits of health research under the U.S. Constitution, there are specific rights to life and liberty that are implicated when women are denied potentially lifesaving interventions or are subjected to potentially lifethreatening risks owing to the lack of appropriate research. Further, the Fifth and Fourteenth Amendments' guarantees of "equal protection" under the law, while not transforming "benefits" into "rights," do treat the distribution of mere "benefits" as a matter of constitutional significance.

    3. Whether or not the benefits are classified as "rights," is there a justification for the disparate treatment, in light of the disparate benefits?

The usual justifications for excluding fertile women from research trials include: male-only data are more homogeneous and therefore more useful; inclusion of women in trials will be unduly costly; government regulation requires the exclusion of women; and the threat to potential fetuses creates a legal and moral imperative to exclude all potentially pregnant women (Merton, V., "The Exclusion of Women from Research Trials," presentation at the Texas Journal of Women and the Law Symposium: New Perspectives on Women, Health and the Law, 5–6 March 1993). Each of these justifications, however, can be shown to be seriously flawed.

Homogeneous data, for example, are only more useful when they adequately serve the purposes for which they are collected. If that purpose is to provide improved therapeutic interventions for men, then current research practices are entirely suitable. If, however, the purpose is to provide improved therapeutic interventions for all persons, then homogeneous data from male-only subject pools are not more useful because they fail to obtain key information needed to decide if the intervention is ready for the market. Similarly, inclusion of women is only "unduly" costly when the cost does not significantly augment the value of the data. Here again, the marginal value of including women is unknown but possibly very high (Report of the Planning Panel of the IOM

Division of Health Sciences Policy, "Issues in the Inclusion of Women in Clinical Trials," 1–2 March 1991). Government policy does at this time limit the full participation of women in research trials. Specifically, Food and Drug Administration (FDA) policy restricts participation of fertile women in Phase I, Phase II, and large-scale Phase III trials, absent certain findings from optional animal research (FDA, "General Considerations for the Clinical Evaluation of Drugs," 1977). Further, Department of Health and Human Services (DHHS) regulations single out pregnant women, and require that research classes be therapeutic only, with minimal risk to the fetus (45 C.F.R. Pt. 46, Subpart B, "Additional Protections Pertaining to Research, Development, and Related Activities Involving Fetuses, Pregnant Women, and Human In Vitro Fertilization").

The exclusion of fertile women from even Phase IV and small-scale Phase III trials, however, as well as the frequent exclusion of all women from Phase I and II trials, testifies to the overbreadth of application of these policies at the level of individual pharmaceutical companies or prinicipal investigators. Further, even the DHHS regulations, which purport to limit the autonomy of pregnant women on behalf of state interests in fetal outcome, are themselves subject to constitutional scrutiny, as they appear to elevate concerns for fetal well-being over concerns for maternal and female well-being.

Although state interest in fetal well-being is certainly permissible (*Planned Parenthood of Southeastern Pennsylvania vs. Casey,* [1992]), it is not superior to a woman's own health and autonomy interests (*In Re A.C.,* 573 A.2d 1235 [D.C. Cir. 1990]) and can even be subordinated to an inchoate desire simply not to have genetic offspring, without implications of bodily autonomy (*Davis v. Davis,* 842 S.W.2d 588 [1992]).

State interests in fetal well-being may increase as viability is achieved (*Roe v. Wade,* 410 U.S.113 [1973]; *Planned Parenthood of Southeastern Pennsylvania v. Casey*). But state interest in previable fetal life, and in preconception potential fetal life, is strictly limited. Even if excluding pregnant women intending to go to term from all nontherapeutic research can be justified on the grounds of fetal protection, excluding all fertile but not currently pregnant women certainly cannot.

4. Does the disparity in benefit operate to disadvantage a protected class of persons? If it does, do the above justifications pass muster?

The Fifth and Fourteenth Amendments to the U.S. Constitution, as mentioned above, require that government actors refrain from denying "equal protection" of the laws under most circumstances. Specifically, where neither the groups suffering the discrimination nor the nature of the discrimination implicates special rights or disadvantaged populations, the discrimination is tolerable as long as there is a rational basis for the government actors' policy. Where, however, fundamental rights are implicated (e.g., the right to marry) or the policy has the purpose or effect of further burdening already disadvantaged classes, the policy is subject to "strict scrutiny" (*United States v. Carolene Products*, 304 U.S. 144 [1938]). Classes of discriminated persons for whom the strict scrutiny standard has been applied include aliens, illegitimate children, and certain racial groups. The theory is that these groups, whether owing to *de jure* impediments (aliens), stigma (illegitimate children), or significant, structural political obstacles (racial minorities), are unable to fully employ the political system and the protections of majoritarian democracy to safeguard their interests. They must therefore be "protected" by the courts from the excesses of the polity.

When strict scrutiny is applied to a governmental policy having the purpose or effect of burdening the exercise of fundamental rights or discriminating against a "protected" class, courts will strike down the policy unless it can be shown that (1) the policy furthers a "compelling" governmental purpose; (2) the purpose is being achieved by the least restrictive means possible; and (3) the policy is narrowly tailored to its goal, neither over- nor underinclusive.

To the extent that excluding fertile women burdens the fundamental rights to life and liberty, these policies are subject to the strict scrutiny test. This is a test they cannot meet. The government's purpose—protection of fetal life and maximization of the cost-effectiveness of research—may well be compelling. But the purpose is not being met by the least restrictive means possible; for example, protection of fetal well-being could be achieved by requiring animal studies on fetotoxicity to precede human studies, and contraception and pregnancy monitoring could be used in human studies.

Further, the policy is both under- and over inclusive. It is underinclusive because it fails to contemplate, let alone address, fetal effects due to paternal exposures. Even if these are predicted to be less common and perhaps less severe than those due to maternal exposure, their complete absence from the policies is unacceptable. It is overinclusive because it excludes many women who, although fertile, are not going to become pregnant, or if pregnant, are not going to carry to term.

If one argues that excluding fertile women does not burden the exercise of a fundamental right, there is still the question of whether the exclusion burdens a "protected" class. Gender discrimination has been held to affect a class—women—who, although historically disadvantaged, do not suffer from the same obstacles as those faced by other "protected" classes. In light of their experience, however, the Supreme Court has deemed them to occupy an "intermediate" status, somewhat like "semi-protected" (*Reed v. Reed*, 404 U.S. 71, 1971) The result is that government policies having the purpose or effect of discriminating against women are accorded an "intermediate" level of judicial review.

Functionally, the Supreme Court has interpreted this to mean that "classifications based on gender must serve important governmental objectives and must be substantially related to the achievement of those objectives" (*Craig v. Boren*, 429 U.S. 190, 1976), or, as stated in a more recent case, the government must have an "exceedingly persuasive justification" (*Mississippi University for Women v. Hogan*, 458 U.S. 718, 1982). Under this analysis, the justifications for excluding fertile women from research are somewhat stronger, but still subject to attack as being ineffective guarantors of fetal well-being and so over inclusive as to fail the test of "substantial relationship" or "exceeding" persuasiveness. It is argued, however, that discrimination against fertile women is not discrimination against women per se. Thus, as fertile women have never achieved even an intermediate protected status in constitutional jurisprudence, the only standard of review applicable to these policies is that of a mere rational relationship between the government interest and its policy.

The question of whether discrimination based upon pregnancy or the capacity to become pregnant is tantamount to gender discrimination has occasioned significant hairsplitting controversy. If government action is gender neutral on its face, e.g., if discrimination based on the capacity to become pregnant is gender neutral because some women, as well as all men, are unable to become pregnant, then despite the discriminatory results of a policy's application, a constitutional violation is demonstrated only if the discrimination is intentional (*Personnel Administrator of Massachusetts v. Feeney*, 442 U.S. 256, 1979).

In the context of employment law, and owing in part to the existence of Title VII's special provisions guaranteeing that pregnant women be treated like nonpregnant women for employment purposes (42 U.S.C. Sec. 2000e(k)), discrimination based on fertility has been held to be equivalent to discrimination based on gender (*U.A.W. v. Johnson Controls*, 111 S. Ct. 1196, 1991). But even compensated service as a research subject would not appear to meet the definition of "employee" under Title VII.

In nonemployment contexts, discrimination based on fertility or pregnancy has frequently been regarded as something distinctly different from discrimination based on gender, despite its obviously disparate impact on male and female populations (*Geduldig v. Aiello*, 417 U.S. 484, 1974; *Michael M. v. Superior Court*, 450 U.S. 464, 1981; *Toomey v. Clark*, 876 F.2d 1433, 9th Cir. 1989; *U.S. v. Flores*, 540 F. 2d 432, 9th Cir. 1976). Under this analysis, once again only a rational relationship must be demonstrated between the discrimination and the government purpose, unless the discrimination is shown to be intentional.

CONCLUSION

To this author, it appears that the exclusion of fertile women from research protocols burdens the fundamental liberty and right to life of fertile women, and functionally burdens the right to life of all women, who are thereby denied the benefits of research on women prior to marketing new drugs and interventions. Thus, a strict scrutiny of the policy would reveal that it is unconstitutional. Alternatively, an argument can be made that discrimination against fertile women, in this context, constitutes discrimination against all women, and thereby must be tested against an intermediate standard of review. Thus, in the context of government controlled research, the Equal Protection Amendment would appear to preclude exclusionary policies because they unconstitutionally deny access to a possibly important benefit to many and possibly most women. Research funded entirely by private means is not similarly covered by the amendment, and even limited receipt of governmental funds may not be sufficient to transform those actions into the sort of "state actions" subject to the amendment (*Rendall-Baker v. Kohn*, 457 U.S. 830, 1982; *Stanturf v. Sipes*, 224 F. Supp. 883, W.D. Mo. 1963; Merton, 1993.) Therefore, this research may well be immune from constitutional challenge.

REFERENCES

Cotton, P. 1990. Is there still too much extrapolation from data on middle-aged white men? *Journal of the American Medical Association* 263:1049.

Society for the Advancement of Women's Health Research (SAWHR) 1991. Toward a women's health research agenda: Findings of the scientific advisory committee. Washington, D.C.: SAWHR.

Levine, R. 1988. Ethics and Regulation of Clinical Research, 2nd ed. New Haven: Yale University Press.

Levi, J. 1991. Unproven AIDS therapies: The Food and Drug Administration and ddI. In: Biomedical Politics, K. Hanna, ed. Washington, D.C.: National Academy Press.

Liability Exposure for Exclusion and Inclusion of Women as Subjects in Clinical Studies

Ellen Flannery and Sanford N. Greenberg

This paper outlines several major issues relating to legal liability for exclusion or inclusion of women as subjects in clinical studies, excluding liability exposure for injury to offspring. The principal focus of the paper is on the testing of pharmaceutical products, because the page constraints make it impossible to cover in depth the issues relating to all types of clinical studies.

The term "clinical studies" encompasses a wide range of activities. In pharmaceutical testing, it usually refers to randomized clinical trials, using either a placebo or an established therapeutic as the control. Clinical studies also include the early-phase safety studies in healthy volunteers, postmarketing studies to expand the indications for use or to investigate safety and effectiveness in special populations (e.g., elderly or children), and investigations of the outcome of health interventions.

Various actors are involved in clinical studies. Companies sponsor studies of pharmaceutical or medical device products; physician investigators conduct and monitor studies; institutional review boards (IRBs) review and approve proposed protocols and informed consent; research institutions provide the study site and may provide attendant medical care; and the Food and Drug Administration (FDA) administers federal statutes and regulations that govern the conduct of clinical investigations, the data required to support product approval applications, and the information contained in product labeling. At least in theory, each of these actors is subject to potential liability for an injury incurred in connection with a clinical study.[1]

It is important to bear in mind that the law is dynamic, not static. New scientific information and new legal theories can quickly change the liability landscape.

One significant change is the way that clinical studies are viewed. Prior to 1981, the focus was on abusive practices in medical research, especially involving women and the elderly, and the need for enhanced protection of human subjects.[2] Now, some commentators assert that participation in clinical trials should be considered a right, especially where the studies involve potentially lifesaving therapies or important research on health outcomes. In considering these different views, recall that some "clinical studies" may involve potentially significant benefits to the participant, while others may involve only sacrifice (e.g., in healthy volunteers) or the element of chance inherent in randomization to a study group. Thus, while inclusion of women in clinical studies may be good for women as a whole, it may or may not be beneficial for the particular women included in a particular study.

TORT LIABILITY DOCTRINES

The actors involved in clinical studies are subject to potential liability in various forms, including product liability lawsuits, medical malpractice actions, or professional licensing board investigations. Even if you are likely to prevail in an action brought against you, the fear of becoming involved in such a legal proceeding is a very strong factor affecting decisions concerning clinical trials. A lawsuit or investigation entails substantial burdens and costs, including the disruption of ongoing work, psychological effects on the individuals who have been accused of causing or contributing to an injury, attorney fees, litigation costs, adverse publicity, and perhaps the costs of settling the plaintiff's claims. Thus, individuals are highly motivated to take the course of action—such as excluding women from a clinical trial—that appears most likely to eliminate or greatly reduce the risk of *becoming involved* in a legal proceeding.

The most significant basis of legal liability for exclusion or inclusion of women as subjects in clinical studies is tort liability.[3] When a plaintiff alleges tortious injury from a drug product, two legal theories are likely to be asserted: negligence and strict liability. In a negligence action, the plaintiff must prove that (1) the defendant (e.g., the manufacturer or investigator) had a legal duty toward the plaintiff, (2) the defendant breached that duty, (3) the plaintiff suffered an injury, and (4) the defendant's breach of its duty was the cause of the plaintiff's injury.[4] In a drug product liability case, the plaintiff would show, for example, that he or she was not given the information that should have been given and that this lack of informed consent caused the plaintiff's injury.

Under strict liability, the manufacturer of a product that is "in a defective condition unreasonably dangerous to the . . . consumer" is subject to liability for injury caused to the consumer without proof of fault by the manufacturer.[5] However, "unavoidably unsafe" products are exempted from this general rule, provided the manufacturer has properly prepared them and has given proper direction and warnings for the products. This exemption (known as the comment k exemption under the Restatement (Second) of Torts § 402A) has been applied by a majority of state courts to prescription drugs and vaccines. Thus, a prescription drug will not be considered unreasonably dangerous if it is accompanied by adequate warnings of potential side effects. Although section 402A expressly applies to sellers of goods, it potentially applies even to those manufacturers who provide investigational drugs free of charge.[6]

Under the so-called learned intermediary doctrine, manufacturers generally can satisfy their duty to warn regarding both prescription drugs and investigational drugs by warning the medical community rather than the ultimate consumer.[7] Warnings are provided through informed consent and the investigator's brochure for investigational products, and through product labeling for marketed products.

The applicability of comment k to prescription drugs varies from state to state. California and Utah have expressly ruled that comment k applies to all properly prepared drugs accompanied by adequate warnings.[8] Wisconsin and Alaska, on the other hand, have refused to adopt comment k and thus declined to protect drug manufacturers from strict liability.[9] The rule in many states is that prescription drugs, prescription medical devices, and vaccines should be accorded the comment k exemption only on a case-by-case basis.[10]

Those states opting for case-by-case application of comment k typically require a drug manufacturer to carry the burden of proving that a product's benefits outweighed its risks at the time of distribution.[11] Often the focus will be on whether a safer, equally efficacious alternative was available when the plaintiff took the challenged product.[12]

Most courts have held that obtaining FDA approval of a drug does not provide a manufacturer with an absolute shield from state tort liability.[13] Evidence of compliance with FDA warning regulations may be introduced as evidence of the adequacy of such warnings.[14] But manufacturers have been held liable for an inadequate warning even where FDA had expressly refused to approve the addition of the warning owing to a lack of evidence supporting causation.[15]

Courts have also held that FDA approval of a vaccine does not preempt state tort claims.[16] Under federal legislation in effect since 1988, however, certain properly prepared childhood vaccines accompanied by adequate warnings to the medical community can be afforded comment k protection, and there is a rebuttable presumption that warnings in compliance with federal regulations are adequate.[17]

The law regarding preemption of state tort claims as to medical devices differs from that applicable to drugs, in large part because of a specific statutory provision for federal preemption of state laws respecting devices (21 U.S.C. § 360k). At least one court has held that any preemptive effects of the Medical Device Amendments (MDA) are not controlling as to IUDs that are classified as drugs as well as devices.[18] Two courts have split on whether the MDA and federal regulations (21 C.F.R. §§ 808.1(b), (d), and part 813) preempt strict liability claims involving experimental intraocular lenses.[19] In recent months, two federal appellate courts have ruled that state claims are preempted for Class III medical devices that require premarket approval of safety and effectiveness by the FDA under 21 U.S.C. § 360c(a)(1)(C).[20] Because these latter decisions were based on express preemption language in the MDA and related federal regulations,[21] their holdings do not extend to drugs, which are approved under statutory provisions with no comparable preemption language (21 U.S.C. § 355).

Clinical investigators, IRBs, and research institutions would be subject to tort liability under negligence principles. As discussed above, this involves showing that the defendant breached a legal duty owed to the plaintiff and the breach caused an injury to the plaintiff. Bases for liability can include violation of a duty imposed by federal regulations, or violation of the standard of care in the community.[22]

LIABILITY FOR EXCLUDING WOMEN FROM CLINICAL STUDIES

Excluding women from clinical trials has long been viewed as a means of avoiding claims for injuries incurred during the studies, especially potential injuries to offspring. This view appears supported by FDA guidelines on conducting clinical studies, which emphasize the exclusion of "women of childbearing potential."[23] Conformance to FDA guidelines is important protection for establishments and individuals, because "use of testing guidelines established by FDA assures acceptance of a test as scientifically valid," and a "guideline may be used in . . . court proceedings to illustrate acceptable and unacceptable procedures or standards."[24] Thus, FDA and other government guidelines on conducting clinical trials can have an important impact on whether women are included or excluded.

An important consideration in reversing the exclusionary approach is its effect on liability after a drug is marketed. If a drug manufacturer fails to include women in a clinical study, it could face a serious risk of liability if postmarketing evidence indicates that the drug is more dangerous or less effective for women than for men. Such evidence might support a claim that the manufacturer had failed adequately to test the product, arguably rendering the product defectively designed. Such evidence also could support a failure-to-warn claim. The law requires manufacturers to warn about not only *known* risks but also *foreseeable* risks that should have been known if the manufacturer had applied "reasonable, developed human skill and foresight."[25] And if the failure to warn of foreseeable risks was due to the deliberate indifference of the manufacturer—for example, the manufacturer tried to avoid learning whether a likely risk was in fact associated with its product—the manufacturer could be liable for punitive damages (intended to punish or deter) as well as for compensatory damages (intended to compensate losses).

Adequate warnings are required even in those states where comment k applies to all prescription drugs. In California a drug manufacturer is responsible for warning of known risks and those that were "reasonably scientifically knowable at the time of distribution."[26] Similarly, under Utah law, drug manufacturers must warn the medical profession of all risks about which they know or should know.[27] Drug manufacturers are deemed to be experts with a continuing duty to keep up with knowledge in their field.[28]

Similar rules apply in those states that afford drugs and vaccines comment k protection on a case-by-case basis. A vaccine can be found defectively designed if it is not "as safe as the best available testing and research permits."[29] Although "unexpected and unknown risks" will not trigger strict liability, sellers are deemed to be experts and are imputed to have all "[k]nowledge of the product's risks based on reliable and obtainable information."[30] To obtain the benefits of comment k, a medical product "must conform to the highest standards of available scientific and technical knowledge."[31] Such standards include state-of-the-art testing of the product.[32]

Drug manufacturers will likely find it increasingly difficult to prove that all-male studies of many drug products constitute state-of-the-art testing. There is growing recognition that the physiological differences between men and women make it scientifically inadequate in many instances to conduct clinical tests or epidemiological studies using only male subjects.[33] For example, in 1990 Dr. Claude Lenfant, Director of the National Heart, Lung, and Blood Institute, responded to a question about the all-male Multiple Risk Factor Intervention Trials—a study of coronary disease risk factors with the ironic acronym "MR. FIT"[34]—by noting the changing views about the adequacy of all-male testing: "In 1972, it was . . . considered appropriate to have a study using only one gender. Today, I would like to submit to you that that would be viewed to be completely inappropriate."[35] And a recent signed editorial in the *Journal of the American Medical Association* commented that "data applicable to elderly patients and to women must be derived from the relevant research source: studies conducted in these specific populations."[36]

IRBs and investigators have an obligation to follow FDA and other governmental regulations and guidelines governing their conduct (e.g., 45 C.F.R. pt. 46). For example, IRBs are responsible for assuring that the "[s]election of subjects is equitable."[37] This regulation might be used as the basis for a claim against an IRB that approves a protocol excluding women. The regulation also identifies pregnant women as one of several "vulnerable populations" that require particular consideration by IRBs.[38] If women are deemed vulnerable under this regulation only when they are pregnant, then non-pregnant women are among the classes that should be equitably selected as subjects for a clinical trial. "Scientific design" is among the factors to be considered when determining "whether the selection of subjects is 'equitable.' "[39] However, the preamble to this regulation as revised in 1991 suggests that it was intended to promote the safety of vulnerable populations more than to assure inclusion of nonvulnerable populations.[40]

In sum, a manufacturer must assure that its clinical trials are adequate to satisfy its two legal obligations—(1) its duty to properly design its drug product, and (2) its duty to provide adequate warnings of known and foreseeable risks. To satisfy these legal obligations, the clinical trials must follow scientifically accepted research methods and include informed consent by the study subjects.

LIABILITY FOR INCLUDING WOMEN IN CLINICAL STUDIES

Federal statutes, regulations, and guidelines governing the conduct of clinical studies are designed to minimize the risks of injury to human subjects. For example, clinical studies of drugs and medical devices must comply with FDA requirements (21 C.F.R. pts. 50, 312, and 812). These include: the submission and approval of a study protocol and informed consent by an IRB; the submission of an application to FDA containing pharmacology and toxicology information from studies in laboratory animals or in vitro showing that it is "reasonably safe" to conduct the proposed clinical investigation, as well as information on previous human experience with the product (e.g., from marketing outside the United States); preparation of an investigator's brochure containing information about the product and its effects, possible risks, and precautions; and prompt reporting by investigators and study sponsors of significant safety information arising during the clinical study.[41] Where all of these requirements have been followed, any injury to a subject that does occur is unlikely to result in liability.

One important question is the extent to which warnings and informed consent permit women to be included in clinical studies in the face of information about either foreseeable risks to women in particular or unknown risks.   An injured subject conceivably could bring an action based on, for example, failure to test in animals for the then unknown effects that resulted in injury. To the extent that any such liability may be imposed, however, it would involve elements of negligence and informed consent that are not gender specific.

Because of their experimental nature, the products involved in clinical studies are especially strong candidates for comment k protection. This point is noted expressly in comment k itself, where it discusses

> new or experimental drugs as to which, because of lack of time and opportunity for sufficient medical experience, there can be no assurance of safety . . . but such experience as there is justifies the marketing and use of the drug notwith-standing a medically recognizable risk.

Provided that the manufacturer warns that the drug is experimental and warns of known and reasonably knowable risks, comment k should apply to an experimental drug.[42] Of course, should evidence of risks to women develop *during* clinical trials, manufacturers would be responsible for determining whether to exclude women from further involvement in the trials as well as to warn about the newly discovered risks.[43]

Investigators testing an experimental drug are likely to be held to the same standards as physicians treating a patient.[44] Thus, a subject's probable theories of recovery would be negligence and lack of informed consent.[45] Federal regulations regarding informed consent prohibit requiring subjects to waive their legal rights.[46] Investigators and institutions conducting clinical trials therefore are potentially liable for negligence in implementing a clinical study.

IRB members also may be sued under state tort law.[47] Although IRBs are not primarily responsible for the design of clinical studies, they potentially could be liable for failing to assure that adequate warnings were given to women where evidence existed of particular risks to women.[48] However, there is apparently no reported case in which IRB members have been successfully sued for breaching their duties to protect research subjects, male or female. The conscientious design and use of informed consent procedures should limit the likelihood that any firm, institution, or individual involved in drug clinical trials would actually be found liable for including women as research subjects.[49]

CONCLUSION

Inclusion of women in clinical studies is unlikely to significantly increase the risk of liability for harm to subjects participating in the clinical trials, while exclusion of women could lead to liability for injuries to women after the product is marketed.

NOTES

1. Federal agencies and employees are protected from suit by the principle of sovereign immunity. The Federal Tort Claims Act provides a limited exception allowing a lawsuit against an agency (not individuals) for injury resulting from negligence in performing "nondiscretionary" acts. 28 U.S.C. §§ 1346(b), 2679, 2680(a). FDA drug regulatory actions pursuant to statute will not be actionable if they involve a permissible exercise of policy discretion. *See Berkovitz v. United States*, 486 U.S. 531 (1988).

2. See *Mink v. University of Chicago*, 460 F. Supp. 713 (N.D. Ill. 1978); FDA Talk Paper T85-30, "Drug Experiments in Nursing Homes" (May 20, 1985).

3. There are other possible causes of action, such as fraud and misrepresentation, see, e.g., *Allen v. G.D. Searle & Co.*, 708 F. Supp. 1142, 1160–61 (D. Or. 1989), and contract related claims, such as breach of warranty, *see, e.g., Castrignano v. E.R. Squibb & Sons, Inc.*, 546 A.2d 775, 783 (R.I. 1988). These are beyond the scope of this paper.

4. See W. Page Keeton et al., *Prosser and Keeton on the Law of Torts* § 30 (5th ed. 1984). See also Restatement (Second) of Torts § 281 (1964).

5. Restatement (Second) of Torts § 402A. Strict liability claims fall into three categories: mismanufacture, design defect, and failure to warn.

6. *See Gaston v. Hunter*, 588 P.2d 326, 338–40 (Ariz. Ct. App. 1978), *review denied* (Ariz. Nov. 21, 1978).

7. *E.g., Grundberg v. Upjohn Co.*, 813 P.2d 89, 97 (Utah 1991) (prescription drug); *Tracy v. Merrell Dow Pharmaceuticals, Inc.*, 569 N.E.2d 875, 879-80 (Ohio 1991) (investigational drug); Gaston, 588 P.2d at 340 (investigational drug). *But cf. Feldman v. Lederle Lab.*, 479 A.2d 374, 388-39 (N.J. 1984) (Feldman I)(indicating that manufacturers may have duty to warn consumers about knowledge of dangers acquired after initial approval and marketing), *rev'd on other grounds after remand*, 561 A.2d 288 (N.J. Super. Ct. App. Div. 1989), rev'd, 592 A.2d 1176 (N.J. 1991) (Feldman II), cert. denied, 112 S. Ct. 3027 (1992). Courts are split about whether the learned intermediary doctrine applies to prescription contraceptives. *Compare, e.g., West v. Searle & Co.*, 806 S.W.2d 608, 614 (Ark. 1991) (yes) with *Odgers v. Ortho Pharmaceutical Corp.*, 609 F. Supp. 867, 878-79 (E.D. Mich. 1985) (no).

8. *Brown v. Superior Court*, 751 P.2d 470, 482-3 & n.11 (Cal. 1988); *Grundberg*, 813 P.2d at 90, 97. Without directly addressing the question of whether comment k applies to all prescription drugs, several other jurisdictions arguably have endorsed such a blanket exemption. *See, e.g., McKee v. Moore*, 648 P.2d 21, 24 (Okla. 1982) (drug manufacturer strictly liable only if it fails to warn physician adequately)

9. *Collins v. Eli Lilly Co.*, 342 N.W.2d 37, 52 (Wis.), cert. denied, 469 U.S. 826 (1984); *Shanks v. Upjohn Co.*, 835 P.2d 1189, 1197-98 (Alaska 1992). While declining to adopt comment k itself, the court in *Shanks* did indicate that drug manufacturers could raise as an affirmative defense to a strict liability design defect claim the type of risk/benefit analysis that many courts use in deciding whether to grant a drug comment k protection. *Id*. at 1196–98.

10. *E.g., West*, 806 S.W.2d at 612 (oral contraceptive); Adams v. G.D. Searle & Co., 576 So. 2d 728, 732-33 (Fla. Dist. Ct. App.) (IUD), *review denied*, 589 So. 2d 290 (Fla. 1991); *Toner v. Lederle Lab.*, 732 P.2d 297, 308 (Idaho 1987) (DPT vaccine);

Savina v. Sterling Drug, Inc., 795 P.2d 915, 924-26 (Kan. 1990) (metrizamide); Pollard v. Ashby, 793 S.W.2d 394, 400 (Mo. Ct. App. 1990) (chymopapain); Feldman I, 479 A.2d at 380, 383 (tetracycline); *Perfetti v. McGhan Med.*, 662 P.2d 646, 650 (N.M. Ct. App.) (mammary prosthesis), *cert. denied*, 662 P.2d 645 (N.M. 1983); *White v. Wyeth Lab., Inc.*, 533 N.E.2d 748, 752 (Ohio 1988) (DPT vaccine); *Castrignano*, 546 A.2d at 781 (DES).

11. *E.g., Toner* 732 P.2d at 306-07.

12. *See, e.g., id.* at 306; *Adams*, 576 So. 2d at 732-33. *But see Harwell v. American Med. Sys.*, 803 F. Supp. 1287, 1297, 1300 (M.D. Tenn. 1992) (under Tennessee law, prescription medical device can be deemed unavoidably unsafe without proof that no safer alternative was available).

13. *E.g., Shanks*, 835 P.2d at 1197 n.10 (Xanax); *Hill v. Searle Lab.*, 884 F.2d 1064, 1068 (8th Cir. 1989) (IUD); *In re Tetracycline Cases*, 747 F. Supp. 543, 550 (W.D. Mo. 1989). See generally Beverly Jacklin, Annotation, *Federal Pre-Emption of State Common-Law Products Liability Claims Pertaining to Drugs, Medical Devices, and Other Health-Related Items*, 98 A.L.R. Fed. 124 (1990).

14. *Savina*, 795 P.2d at 931; *Feldman II*, 592 A.2d at 1197.

15. *Wooderson v. Ortho Pharmaceutical Corp.*, 681 P.2d 1038 (Kan.), *cert. denied*, 469 U.S. 965 (1984).

16. *E.g., Toner*, 732 P.2d at 311 n.12; *Abbot v. American Cyanamid Co.*, 844 F.2d 1108, 1112-14 (4th Cir.), *cert. denied*, 488 U.S. 908 (1988). *But cf. Hurley v. Lederle Lab.*, 863 F.2d 1173, 1179 (5th Cir. 1988) (preemption of inadequate warning claim).

17. 42 U.S.C. §§ 300aa-22(b), (c) (1988); *see* H.R. Rep. No. 100-391 (I), 100th Cong., 1st Sess. 691 (1987); *Abbot*, 844 F.2d at 1117 (Wilkins, J., concurring).

18. *Allen*, 708 F. Supp. at 1150-52.

19. *Compare Slater v. Optical Radiation Corp.*, 961 F.2d 1330, 1333 (7th Cir.) (defective design claim preempted), *cert. denied*, 113 S. Ct. 327 (1992) *with Mitchell v. Iolab Corp.*, 700 F. Supp. 877, 878-79 (E.D. La. 1988) (no preemption) (*appeal pending*).

20. *Stamps v. Collagen Corp.*, No. 92-2084 (5th Cir. Feb. 19, 1993); *King v. Collagen Corp.*, No. 92-1278 (1st Cir. Jan. 15, 1993). *Cf. Moore v. Kimberly-Clark*, 867 F.2d 243, 246-47 (5th Cir. 1989) (holding that failure-to-warn and labeling claims were preempted for Class II device, which does not require premarket approval, but defective construction and design claims not preempted). *But cf. Larsen v. Pacesetter Sys., Inc.*, 837 P.2d 1273, 1282 (Haw. 1992) (declining to find preemption regarding a Class III device that underwent a less rigorous premarket approval process than the devices involved in the *Collagen* cases because the *Larsen* device was " 'substantially equivalent' " to devices already approved for marketing).

21. *See Stamps*, slip op. at 6-8 and n.1; *King*, slip op. at 8-10.

22. *E.g., Gaston*, 588 P.2d at 346, 350-51. Depending on state law, specialists may be held to a national standard of care. *See id.* at 346. If an investigator were deemed a specialist, the investigator would be held to " 'the standard of care required of physicians in the same specialty. . . .' " *Id.* (quoting *Kronke v. Danielson*, 499 P.2d 156, 159 (Ariz. 1972)). A physician/investigator's responsibilities include obtaining the subject's informed consent. *Id.* at 350-51.

23. FDA, *General Considerations for the Clinical Evaluation of Drugs* 10 (September 1977) (DHEW/FDA Pub. 77-3040).

24. 21 C.F.R. § 10.90(b)(1)(ii) and (8) (1992).

25. Restatement (Second) of Torts § 402A comment j. *See, e.g., Shanks*, 835 P.2d at 1200 (indicating that, under strict liability failure-to-warn claim, the defendant must "prove that the risk was scientifically unknowable at the time the product was distributed to the plaintiff"); *Feldman I*, 479 A.2d at 388 (similar).

26. *Brown*, 751 P.2d at 483.

27. *Grundberg*, 813 P.2d at 97. *See also Enright* v. *Eli* Lilly & Co., 568 N.Y.S.2d 550, 556 (drug manufacturers are not immune "from liability stemming from their failure to conduct adequate research and testing prior to the marketing of their products") (dictum), *cert. denied*, 112 S. Ct. 197 (1991).

28. *Grundberg*, 813 P.2d at 98.

29. *Toner*, 732 P.2d at 306.

30. *Id.* at 307 (citing *Feldman I*, 479 A.2d at 386-87; *Belle Bonfils Memorial Blood Bank* v. *Hansen*, 665 P.2d 118, 126 (Colo. 1983)).

31. *Belle Bonfils*, 665 P.2d at 126.

32. *See id.* at 125, 127. *Cf. Feldman I*, 479 A.2d at 386-87 (indicating that drug manufacturers may have duty to continue testing after product first approved). The value of having an extensive data base regarding a drug's safety when defending against product liability actions is suggested in *Daubert v. Merrell Dow Pharmaceuticals, Inc.*, 951 F.2d 1128, 1129 (9th Cir. 1991) (noting defendant's citation of "30 published studies involving over 130,000 patients"), *cert. granted*, 113 S. Ct. 320 (1992).

33. *See, e.g.*, Jean Hamilton (ed.), Clinical Pharmacology Panel Report 1, *in* Susan J. Blumenthal et al. (eds.), *Forging a Women's Health Research Agenda*, Conference Proceedings, National Women's Health Resource Center (Washington, D.C. October 1991) ("Despite the lack of systematic study in the past, clinically significant sex, hormone or gender-related effects have been reported for the following drugs or types of drugs: antidepressants (e.g., lithium), antidopaminergic antipsychotics, anticonvulsants (e.g. phenytoin), an antihypertensive (propranolol), several sedative-hypnotics (e.g., diazepam; methaqualone), alcohol, and possibly for insulin, synthetic glucocorticoids, theophylline, and caffeine. A 'clinically significant effect' is that having implications for altering decisions about pharmacotherapy for women, not just findings that reach statistical significance.")

34. *NIH Reauthorization and Protection of Health Facilities: Hearings Before the Subcomm. on Health and the Environment of the House Comm. on Energy and Commerce*, 101st Cong., 2d Sess. 237 (1990) (testimony of Rep. Snowe).

35. *Id.* at 286. Other observers have questioned a study of the long-term use of aspirin to help prevent myocardial infarction because the study involved only men and left unclear whether the benefits observed for men would apply to women as well. *See, e.g.*, L. Elizabeth Bowles, *The Disfranchisement of Fertile Women in Clinical Trials: The Legal Ramifications of and Solutions for Rectifying the Knowledge Gap*, 45 Vand. L. Rev. 877, 887-88 (1992). Although later studies indicated an apparent beneficial effect for women, *see id.* at 888 (citing Lawrence Appel and Trudy Bush, *Preventing Heart Disease in Women: Another Role for Aspirin*, 266 *JAMA* 565 (1991)); *NIH Reauthorization: Hearings Before the Subcomm. on Health and the Environment of the House Comm. on Energy and Commerce*, 102d Cong., 1st Sess. 233 (1991) (testimony of Dr. Bernardine Healy), the Director of the National Institutes of Health, Dr. Bernardine

Healy, acknowledged as recently as 1991 that it was still unclear whether "aspirin poses a unique danger for women." *Id.* Dr. Healy indicated opposition to proposed legislation that would have required the inclusion of women in NIH-sponsored clinical studies absent a showing that such inclusion was inappropriate. *See id.* at 232. She noted, however, that similar guidelines were already NIH policy and that the proposed legislation thus was not necessary. *Id.*

    36. Nanette K. Wenger, *Exclusion of the Elderly and Women from Coronary Trials: Is Their Quality of Care Compromised?* 268 *JAMA* 1460, 1461 (1992). Because elderly Americans are disproportionately women, age-based exclusions tend to screen out women. *See* Jerry H. Gurwitz et al., *The Exclusion of the Elderly and Women from Clinical Trials in Acute Myocardial Infarction,* 268 *JAMA* 1417, 1419-20 (1992). Such exclusion has created "profound confusion for the practitioner" regarding appropriate therapy for elderly patients. *Id.* at 1421.

    37. 21 C.F.R. § 56.111(a)(3) (1992).

    38. *Id.*

    39. 46 Fed. Reg. 8958, 8969 (1981).

    40. *See* 56 Fed. Reg. 28025, 28027 (1991). *But cf.* 56 Fed. Reg. 28003, 28010 (1991) (discussing similar provision in Federal Policy for the Protection of Human Research Subjects: "In exercising their responsibilities, IRBs are charged with evaluating the *benefits and the burdens* of the research. . . .") (emphasis added).

    41. *E.g.,* 21 C.F.R. §§ 312.23, 312.32 (1992).

    42. *See Gaston,* 588 P.2d at 340. *See also Toner,* 732 P.2d at 307 (noting comment k's specific discussion of experimental drugs).

The *Gaston* court also declined to treat drug experiments as abnormally dangerous activities and thus refused to impose the even harsher regime of absolute liability on either investigators or manufacturers. 588 P.2d at 341-42. The court based its decision in part on the rationale that the law regarding absolute liability does not apply to those who voluntarily engage in the activity. *Id.* at 341. *See also Whitlock v. Duke Univ.,* 637 F. Supp. 1463, 1475-76 (M.D.N.C. 1986) (rejecting similar claim in case involving non-therapeutic experiment), *aff'd per curiam,* 829 F.2d 1340 (4th Cir. 1987).

    43. *See, e.g., Feldman I,* 479 A.2d at 386-87.

    44. *E.g., Gaston,* 588 P.2d at 346, 350-51.

    45. *See, e.g., Valenti v. Prudden,* 397 N.Y.S.2d 181 (App. Div. 1977) (prison inmate voluntarily involved in non-therapeutic surgical experiment brought claims for negligence and lack of informed consent against hospital and doctor). *See also Anderson v. George H. Lanier Memorial Hosp.,* 1993 U.S. App. LEXIS 2161, at *18-20 (11th Cir. Feb. 12, 1992) (although related malpractice claims were barred by statute of limitation, hospital at which investigational devices installed is potentially liable for fraud due to physician's alleged failure to obtain informed consent); *Friter v. Iolab Corp.,* 607 A.2d 1111 (Pa. Super. 1992) (hospital conducting clinical study of investigational device can be held liable for battery and failure to assure that physician obtained informed consent required under federal regulations; plaintiff had already settled with physician's representatives). *Cf. Tracy,* 569 N.E.2d at 879-80 (holding that learned intermediary rule applies in investigational context when investigator determines subject's suitability for inclusion and monitors subject's involvement). Because the *Tracy* court focussed on whether the investigator acted as a *treating* physician would, there is some question

whether its holding would apply in cases involving subjects whose involvement in a clinical trial was entirely *non*-treatment oriented.

46. 21 C.F.R. § 50.20 (1992).

47. *See* 46 Fed. Reg. 8958, 8961 (1981).

48. *See generally id.* ("[T]he primary responsibilities of an IRB are to assure that human subjects are adequately protected, are not exposed to unnecessary risks, and are provided with enough information about a study so that they can give effective informed consent. However, the agency believes that it is impossible to divorce completely considerations of science from those of ethical acceptability and of protection of human subjects. Some type of scientific review is necessary to determine whether the risk to which subjects are exposed is reasonable.")

49. *See, e.g., id.*

Liability Exposure When Offspring Are Injured Because of Their Parents' Participation in Clinical Trials

Ellen Wright Clayton

The exclusion of fertile men and women, and more particularly pregnant women, from clinical trials is often justified on the basis that fetuses must be protected and that if fetuses are injured, the potential liability will be too great. Both of these arguments are fundamentally flawed. Looking first just from the child's perspective, the earlier the teratogenic or mutagenic effects of drugs are detected, the fewer children will be exposed. From the perspective of investigators and particularly of the manufacturers whose interventions are being tested, the risk of incurring liability during the early stages of drug investigation is actually quite small whereas the potential for substantial liability is much greater once a fetotoxic drug enters widespread use.

Does the desire of the federal government to include women in clinical trials preempt claims alleging the children were injured as a result? A threshold question is whether children and their parents can bring tort claims at all because permitting such claims works counter to the federal purpose. The argument here is that if there is a threat of liability, efforts to include women in clinical trials will fail because potential parents will not enroll in and third parties will not include potential parents in clinical trials. The majority's dictum on *Johnson Controls* that the goal of Title VII of ensuring equal access to the work place could preempt tort claims brought by children allegedly injured by their mothers' exposure to lead in the work place would appear to support this line of reasoning.[1] Yet when directly confronted with defining the scope of preemption in 1992, the Supreme Court made clear that it will not find preemption unless there is a direct conflict between state and federal law or unless Congress clearly intended to occupy the field completely.[2] These conditions are only rarely met. In the area of drug research, for example, no appellate court has found that the extensive federal regulation of the information contained in package inserts and the *Physicians' Desk Reference* totally preempts state tort claims alleging inadequate warning.[3] Further, there is no evidence that Congress intends to eliminate claims by later-born children in order to ensure that potential parents be included in clinical trials, so it is unlikely that courts will find that these tort claims are preempted.

Identifying potential claimants and their claims. Assuming that tort claims are not preempted, defining the types of claims that can be brought following the ingestion of a fetotoxic drug becomes important because the potential claims vary widely and lead to very different measures of damages. The two most important factors in this analysis are whether the child was born alive and what the parents would have done had they known about the risk. Claims can be brought on behalf of children only if they were born alive.[4] When children are born alive and when their parents allege that they would not have taken the drug had they known about the risk of fetotoxic effects, children can assert claims for prenatal injury, saying that they could otherwise have been born healthy. In recent years, most courts have looked favorably on prenatal injury claims and on occasion have awarded very large amounts of damages, commensurate with the child's special needs over the course of a lifetime.[5] By contrast, children are said to be seeking damages for "wrongful life" when they are born alive but their parents say that more information would have led them to avoid childbearing. These claims have almost universally been rejected by courts and legislatures.[6] Interestingly, one court permitted two children who were born with fetal hydantoin syndrome to recover some damages for wrongful life when their mother alleged that she had expressed concern about taking Dilantin during pregnancy to her providers, who inappropriately reassured her that there was little risk.[7]

The nature of parents' claims differs depending on whether the child was born alive or not and on whether the parents would have avoided the drug or put off procreation. When the children were live-born and the parents say they would not have taken the drug, the parents may recover the medical expenses not covered by the child's claims. In most cases, however, the parents will not receive damages for their own emotional pain and suffering because they are seen as bystanders to their child's injury. Even in the jurisdictions that are most sympathetic to parents' claims for emotional injury, parents must allege that they were aware at the time of the child's injury that the defendant's actions were responsible, conditions that can probably never be met for injuries caused by fetotoxic drugs.[8]

If the parents have a live child but assert that they would have avoided childbearing had they known more, their claim is one for "wrongful birth." Courts have generally permitted at least some aspects of the parents' claims, although some legislatures have limited these causes of action.[9] These claims, when permitted, can also support large damage awards.

When a child is stillborn as a result of negligence, some jurisdictions permit the beneficiaries of the fetus' estate—usually the parents—to bring an action for wrongful death,[10] although some states require that the fetus be viable at the time the lethal injury occurred.[11] Many other states, however, refuse to permit such claims at all.[12] Even when these claims are permitted, however, the amount of damages is usually relatively small.

Children's claims against their parents. The next question is who can be sued. Whether children injured by drugs can sue the parent who took them turns, first of all, on the law of parent–child immunity in the state where the family resides. States generally have begun to limit this sort of immunity: some never had it or got rid of it altogether; others have declared that only some decisions by parents may give rise to liability. Yet a few states retain complete immunity.[13] Three states have specifically addressed children's claims that they were injured by their mothers' behavior during pregnancy. Two states permitted the children's claims,[14] including one case in which the child alleged that he was injured when his mother took tetracycline while she was pregnant. One state denied a child a cause of action,[15] saying that allowing the claim would intrude too deeply into the lives of pregnant women.

In the states that have struck down parent–child tort immunity in whole or in part, the next issue is what sort of parental behavior will give rise to liability. At the least, parents must be negligent, that is, their choices must be ones that other reasonable people would not have made, before they can be held liable. The factors that should enter into that calculus include the general deference we give to patients in choosing their treatment,[16] the seriousness of the parent's medical problem, and the availability of nonfetotoxic alternatives. Parents' choices would probably be found acceptable in most situations. It would probably be reasonable, for example, to choose chemotherapy with powerful mutagens for treatment of cancer. It might be less reasonable, by contrast, for a woman of childbearing years to use ACE inhibitors which are known teratogens to treat hypertension when there are other nonfetotoxic options available.

If the parent's decision to take the research drug was not negligent, the final argument that might be made by a child is that the parent was unreasonable or negligent in deciding to have the child. Such "wrongful life" claims by children are highly disfavored in general, as was discussed above, but they are particularly unlikely to succeed when made against parents.[17]

Impact of one parent's negligence on the other parent's claims. This issue has most commonly been litigated in the context of wrongful death, but the analysis is applicable as well to claims for wrongful birth or the ancillary claims to prenatal injury. In general, a potential beneficiary may not recover damages if his or her negligence caused the wrongful death, but the negligence of one beneficiary does not preclude recovery by other beneficiaries.[18] One court recently held that the father of a child stillborn because of the mother's negligence could not recover damages because the mother might indirectly benefit.[19] This imputation of the negligence of one parent to the other, however, has been criticized as a "senseless survival of a discarded concept of marital unity."[20] Thus, if one parent negligently takes a fetotoxic drug in a jurisdiction that permits wrongful death actions when children are stillborn, the other parent may well be able to recover damages.

Claims against third parties. Although children may be able to sue their parents for taking part in a clinical trial, the public debate about the desirability of including fertile and pregnant individuals in clinical trials is much more heavily influenced by the fear that injured children will sue third parties, including the researcher/physician who provided the drug, the institution in which the research occurred, and the drug manufacturer. The basic rules of negligence and strict liability are discussed at length in this volume's paper by Flannery and Greenberg.[21] Claims on behalf of children, however, present some special issues since they did not directly consent to the intervention. For purposes of this discussion, we can group the possible bases of liability into two groups—one for lack of warning of possible fetotoxic effects, based in the law of informed consent or duty to warn in strict liability; and the other for problems with the intervention itself or the way it was administered, based in the rules governing defective products or negligence.

Cases in which parents were not warned are in some ways easier. If the parent says that she was not told of the potential fetotoxic effects of the drug, then the child and parents may be able to pursue claims against researchers and the health care institutions in which they work for prenatal injury and economic/emotional injury or wrongful life and wrongful birth, depending on whether the parent would have avoided taking the drug or decided against childbearing. Claims against manufacturers, however, may be barred by the learned intermediary doctrine.

Courts have not confronted a case in which the parents say that they knew at the time they took the drug about its potential effects on their unborn child, even though this situation is likely to occur in research because of the stringent federal requirements for disclosure. In this setting, although the law is by no means clear, the distinction between the two types of claims is critical. If the parents were adequately informed, the child who was injured prenatally probably cannot be heard to complain that he or she would not have agreed to the exposures. Fetuses or preconceptuses cannot be warned, and as Professor Merton demonstrated, parents can consent to some types of nontherapeutic research for children who are already born.[22] Prospective parents should have even greater latitude to "choose" nontherapeutic research on their unborn children, particularly when the protocol offers potential benefit to the parent who is enrolled. There may, however, be settings in which third parties are not entitled to rely on even the fully informed consent of prospective parents to immunize them from later liability if the protocol poses very serious risks to the unborn child while offering little benefit to the subject adult or to adults in general.

A different problem arises when the intervention was provided negligently or was defective. In that setting, as was mentioned by Justice White in *Johnson Controls*,[23] many cases hold that parents cannot anticipatorily release their children's potential claims.[24] If even documents clearly designated as releases do not preclude children's claims, then a parent's signature on a document for informed consent to research involving a potentially fetotoxic drug would not bar the injured child's suit. One might argue that cases rejecting anticipatory releases, which often deal with potential liability for recreational activities, do not apply to the more complex decisions of a potential parent to take a drug that may help him or her at the risk of harm to future children. This argument may not prevail because the rule barring parental releases of children's claims is based in part on the desire to avoid conflicts of interest between parents and children, which is exactly the problem posed by parental use of potentially fetotoxic drugs. Finally, even if parents can release some claims, releases are strictly construed and therefore must be clearly written, especially where they purport to waive claims for future negligence.

Another potential barrier confronting children in this setting is the argument that the parent's consent acts as a superseding cause that shields the researcher or manufacturer from liability. The line of reasoning should be rejected on the grounds that the parent's agreement to use the drug is a clearly foreseeable result of the efforts to test it and that permitting this defense would vitiate the ban on parental releases.[25]

Does it matter whether the researcher works for the government? The states vary widely in whether they allow physicians who work for governmental institutions and the institutions themselves to be sued. Some states say that provision of health care is not protected because it is not inherently governmental or because the state does not exercise control over the provider,[26] while others waive immunity to the extent of available insurance coverage.[27] Some states, however, retain immunity for some providers and government institutions.[28] Under the Federal Tort Claims Act, physicians who are working within the scope of their employment for the federal government may not be sued in their individual capacities. The federal government can be sued for some of its employees' torts, including medical malpractice and lack of informed consent, but not for battery.[29]

May children sue the federal government if they were injured before birth by their parent's participation in research while enlisted in the armed services? In *Feres v. United States*,[30] the Supreme Court held that an injured serviceman cannot bring a tort action against the government for claims incident to service. Subsequently, a number of cases held that claims on behalf of fetuses harmed by negligent prenatal care of women who were members of the military were barred by the *Feres* doctrine.[31] These courts reasoned that medical care was incident to service and that if the service member cannot sue, the child cannot sue for any derivative injuries.[32] Recent cases, however, have ruled to the contrary, challenging both of these lines of argument. First, some cases have held that the children injured by negligent prenatal care to a service member are suing for their own injuries and not asserting simply derivative claims.[33] Second, a recent and potentially more far-reaching case has challenged the notion that all injuries resulting from medical care are "incident to service." A service woman was allowed to pursue a claim for injuries sustained as a result of her voluntary participation in a military-run blood donor drive on the grounds that her donation did not implicate sensitive military matters and was more civilian in nature.[34] Thus, while children injured as a result of their parents' participation as members of armed services in clinical research are still unlikely to succeed in their claims against the federal government, these recent trends raise the possibility that their claims soon will be more successful.

The risk of liability for injuries incurred during research is low. Looked at simply from the perspectives of legal doctrine and of the extensive disclosure that typically occurs in the research setting, then, there will rarely be any basis for successful lawsuits by children or particularly by parents. In addition, as a practical matter, there are a very small number of cases alleging injuries incurred during research. Perhaps subjects do not sue because they feel that they somehow "assumed the risk," even though the law no longer accepts this notion as a defense to tort claims. Perhaps the small number of suits is part of the phenomenon that the overwhelming majority of people injured by medical malpractice do not pursue claims.[35] But the result of all these theoretical and practical limitations is that the risk that researchers, institutions, or manufacturers will be held liable for large amounts of money for injuries children suffer as a result of their parents' participation in clinical trials is actually quite low.

The potential for liability is much greater if efforts are not made to detect fetotoxic effects. Here it is useful to compare the situation of a manufacturer of a drug that was in widespread use while its teratogenic effects were unknown but knowable with that of a manufacturer of a known teratogen. In the former case, many children may be injured and their lawyers may argue that the manufacturer had a duty to find out about these effects. As Flannery and Greenberg have suggested, this argument is likely to meet with increasing success, particularly in light of growing pressure to include fertile people in trials; and where it is accepted, it could lay the basis for tremendous liability. Physicians, too, would face potential liability if they did not warn their patients about the lack of data or failed to notice early reports in the literature. Both manufacturers and physicians would also face the prospect of having issues of causation decided in the crucible of the courtroom, where the scientific method is but one factor in the determination.

By contrast, the manufacturer of a known teratogen can transfer the risk of liability to the health care provider under the learned intermediary doctrine by promulgating a sufficiently stringent warning about the fetotoxic effects.[36] The provider, in turn, can avoid liability by choosing another nonfetotoxic alternative. Where an appropriate alternative is not available, the provider can decrease or eliminate his or her exposure by telling patients about the potential risks and allowing them to share or shoulder the responsibility.

Finding out about fetotoxicity averts harm to children. Even though the children injured by thalidomide and DES have not often succeeded in their efforts to obtain compensation from drug manufacturers,[37] they were nonetheless harmed because their mothers took these drugs. The legal system may shift some of the costs of injuries away from the injured parties, but the uncompensated harms do not go away. It is also possible that children are currently being injured by their parents' ingestion of drugs whose fetotoxic effects have not yet been detected. Finally, it is clear that having this information alters behavior in ways that minimize children's exposure—physicians usually will not prescribe fetotoxic drugs and fertile individuals usually will not choose to take them. It may be that most fetotoxic effects will not be detected in clinical trials. But unless the drug will never be used in fertile individuals, the answer to this dilemma is not to exclude such people from clinical trials but rather to broaden the scope of inquiry to require animal studies of mutagenicity and teratogenicity prior to testing or at least marketing for human use and to implement truly effective methods of long-term surveillance that begin during clinical trials.

In closing, since information obtained during research will benefit future children, proposals to limit or ban liability for children injured while the data are being collected seem unjust unless support were otherwise provided for their medical and other needs. Simply to ban claims would mean that the children injured by research and their families would bear all the costs while potential parents and other children receive all the benefits. In the end, the costs of potential liability to children injured as a result of their parents' participation in clinical trials may simply be ones that must be borne as costs of ensuring that new products are fully tested before they are brought to market.

***

I would like to thank Carrie Genova for her excellent research assistance and Jay Clayton and Nicholas S. Zeppos for their helpful comments on earlier drafts.

NOTES

1. International Union, UAW v Johnson Controls, 111 S.Ct. 1196, 1208–09 (1991).
2. Cippolone v. Liggett Group, Inc., 112 S.Ct. 2608 (1992).
3. Abbot v. American Cyanamid Co., 844 F.2d 1108 (4th Cir.), cert. denied, 488 U.S. 908 (1988); *see also* Reeder v. Hammond, 336 N.W.2d 3 (Mich. App. 1983)(summary judgment for defendant on issue of warning not warranted in light of physician's testimony that warning regarding potential teratogenicity of Biphetamine was inadequate); *cf.,* Hurley v. Lederle Laboratories, 863 F.2d 1173 (5th Cir. 1988)(can argue that manufacturer withheld information from FDA).
4. Children's claims are typically tolled, which means that the statute of limitations does not begin to run, during their minority. Some states have passed statutes limiting this period, but where the traditional rule still applies, children injured prior to birth can bring claims until they are twenty years old. *See* Renslow v. Mennonite Hosp., 367 N.E.2d 1250 (Ill. 1977). Thus, when time has passed, the child may still be able to sue even when the parents's potential claims are barred.
5. W. Page Keeton, et al. Prosser and Keeton on the Law of Torts § 55, 367 (5th ed. 1984).
6. Ellen Wright Clayton, *What the Law Says About Reproductive Genetic Testing—and What It Doesn't,* in Women and Reproductive Genetic Testing: The Dilemmas of Reproductive Decision Making (K.Rothenberg, E. Thomson, eds.) in press, 1993.
7. Harbeson v. Parke-Davis, Inc., 656 P.2d 483 (Wash. 1983).
8. *Compare* Vaccaro v. Squibb, 418 N.E.2d 386 (NY 1980)(parents can recover only when they were in "zone of danger") *with* Ochoa v. Superior Ct., 703 P.2d 1 (Cal. 1985)(more permissive jurisdiction). *But see* Romero v. U.S., 954 F.2d 223 (4th Cir. 1992)(permitting such a claim as part of consequential damages). This analysis assumes that the drugs caused no direct personal injury to the parents. If the parents did have such an injury, they are able to recover fully for emotional pain and suffering, no matter what its source.
9. *Supra* note 6.

10. *E.g.,* Volk v. Baldazo, 651 P.2d 11 (Idaho 1982); Mone v. Greyhound Lines, 331 N.E.2d 916 (Mass. 1975).

11. *E.g.,* O'Grady v. Brown, 654 S.W.2d 904 (Mo. 1983).

12. *E.g.,* Justus v. Atchison, 565 P.2d 122 (Cal. 1977); Endresz v. Friedberg, 248 N.E.2d 901 (N.Y. 1969); *see generally* Keeton et al, *supra* note 5, at 55, 369–370, nn. 31 & 32.

13. Cates v. Cates, 588 N.E.2d 330, 334–335 (Ill. App.), app. granted, 602 N.E.2d 448 (Ill. 1992)(listing cases).

14. Grodin v. Grodin, 301 N.W.2d 869 (Mich. App. 1981); Bonte v. Bonte, 616 A.2d 464 (N.H. 1992).

15. Stallman v. Youngquist, 531 N.E.2d 355 (Ill. 1988).

16. In In re AC, 573 A.2d 1235 (DC Ct App 1990) (en banc), the Court of Appeals implicitly affirmed the appropriateness of the pregnant woman's decisions to have some intervention for her own comfort in the terminal stages of her illness even though they posed some additional risk to her fetus.

17. Only one court has said in dicta that a child with a genetic disorder could sue his parents if they chose to carry him to term. Curlender v. Bio-Sciences Labs, 165 Cal. Rptr. 477 (Cal. App. 1980). The California legislature almost immediately passed a law providing that children cannot sue their parents for "wrongful life." Cal. Health & Safety Code § 43.6 (West 1991).

18. Nudd v. Matsoukas, 131 N.E.2d 525 (Ill. 1956); Shinauer v. Szymanski, 471 N.E.2d 477 (Ohio 1984).

19. Chamness v. Fairtrace, 511 N.E.2d 839 (Ill. App.) app den., 515 N.E.2d 103 (Ill. 1987)

20. Keeton et al, *supra* note 5, at § 127, 959, n.57.

21. Ellen J. Flannery & Sanford N. Greenberg, *Liability Exposure for Exclusion and Inclusion of Women as Subjects in Clinical Studies,* this volume.

22. Vanessa Merton, *The Impact of Current Relevant Federal Regulations on the Inclusion of Female Subjects in Clinical Studies,* this volume; 45 C.F.R. § 46.406.

23. *Supra* note 1, at 1211 & n.3 (White, J., concurring).

24. *E.g.,* Apicella v. Valley Forge Military Academy, 630 F. Supp. 20 (E.D. Pa. 1985); Fedor v. Mauwehu Council, Boy Scouts of America, 143 A.2d 466 (Conn. Super. 1958); Doyle v Bowdoin College, 403 A.2d 1206 (Me. 1979); Fitzgerald v. Newark Morning Ledger Co., 267 A.2d 557 (NJ Super 1970); Childress v. Madison County, 777 S.W.2d 1 (Tenn. App. 1989), cert. denied; Scott v. Pacific West Mountain Resort, 834 P.2d 6 (Wash. 1992).

25. Keeton et al, *supra* note 5, at § 44, 301–311.

26. Gleason v. Beesinger, 708 F. Supp. 157 (S.D. Tex. 1989); Gould v. O'Bannon, 770 S.W.2d 220 (Ky. 1989); James v. Jane, 282 S.E.2d 864 (Va. 1980).

27. Poss v. Georgia Regional Hosp., 676 F. Supp. 258 (S.D. Ga. 1987), aff'd, 874 F.2d 820 (11th Cir.), cert. denied, 493 U.S. 850 (1989); Bly v. Young, 732 S.W.2d 157 (Ark. 1987).

28. Hyde v. Univ. Mich. Board Regents, 393 N.W.2d 847 (Mich. 1986); Gargiulo v. Ohar, 387 S.E.2d 787 (Va. 1990)(fellow who injured patient in course of research was immune because of state's interest in training specialists).

29. 28 U.S.C.A. §§ 2674–2680 (West 1992); Keir v. U.S., 853 F.2d 398 (6th Cir. 1988); Supchak v. U.S., 365 F.2d 844 (3d Cir. 1966).

30. 340 U.S. 135 (1950). A later case extended this immunity to injuries incurred while participating voluntarily in a military experiment. U.S. v. Stanley, 483 U.S. 669 (1987).

A health care provider acting within the scope of his employment in the military may not be sued independently for malpractice. 10 U.S.C.A. § 1089 (West 1992); U.S. v. Smith, 111 S.Ct. 1180 (1991).

31. Irvin v. U.S., 845 F.2d 126 (6th Cir.), cert. denied, 488 U.S. 975 (1988); *cf.*, Scales v. U.S., 685 F.2d 970 (5th Cir. 1982), cert. denied, 460 U.S. 1082 (1983)(child born with congenital rubella syndrome because mother negligently given rubella vaccine while pregnant).

32. Mondelli v. U.S., 711 F.2d 567 (3d Cir. 1983), cert. denied, 465 U.S. 1021 (1984); Lombard v. U.S., 690 F.2d 215 (D.C. Cir. 1982), cert. denied, 462 U.S. 1118 (1983); Monaco v. U.S. 661 F.2d 129 (9th Cir. 1981), cert. denied, 456 U.S. 989 (1982).

33. These courts reason that the child injured in utero is in the same position as the civilian dependent injured by the negligence of military personnel whose claims are not barred by *Feres*. They vary, however, in their receptiveness to parents' claims. Romero v. U.S., 954 F.2d 223 (4th Cir. 1992)(parents allowed to pursue claims for "loss of filial love, mental anguish, and the financial burden for Joshua's physical condition" as well); Del Rio v. U.S., 833 F.2d 282 (11th Cir. 1987)(however, mother's claim for wrongful death of one twin barred by *Feres*); Graham v. U.S., 753 F. Supp. 994 (D. Me. 1990)(parents' claims waived).

34. Johnson v. U.S., 735 F. Supp. 1 (D.D.C. 1990), mot. denied, partial summary jment granted, 1993 U.S. Dist. LEXIS 137 (D.D.C. 1993). She alleged that she was incorrectly told that she was HIV positive which led her to have an abortion she otherwise would not have had.

35. Patients, Doctors, and Lawyers: Medical Injury, Malpractice Litigation, and Patient Compensation in New York: The Report of the Harvard Medical Practice Study to the State of New York. 1990; JS Kakalik, NM Pace, Costs and Compensation Paid in Tort Litigation. 1986.

36. Bealer v Hoffman-La Roche, Inc., 729 F. Supp. 43 (ED La 1990); Hunt v Hoffman-LaRoche, Inc., 785 F. Supp. 547 (D. Md. 1992); Felix v. Hoffman-La Roche, Inc., 540 So.2d 102 (Fla. 1989); *see generally* Salmon v. Parke Davis, 520 F.2d 1359 (4th Cir. 1975); McDaniel v. McNeil Laboratories, 241 N.W.2d 822 (Neb. 1976).

37. Elizabeth L. Bowles, *The Disenfranchisement of Fertile Women in Clinical Trials: The Legal Ramifications of and Solutions for Rectifying the Knowledge Gap*, 45 Vand. L. Rev. 877 (1992).

Compensation for Research Injuries

Wendy K. Mariner

I have been asked to discuss the advantages and disadvantages of alternative ways to (1) limit liability for sponsors of research and (2) compensate research subjects, when women are used as subjects of research. This definition of the subject seems loaded with assumptions: first, that liability is interfering with important research that will benefit women; and second, that women research subjects, or their future children, will suffer great harm as a result of research.

These two assumptions do not coexist comfortably. If liability is preventing sponsors from doing research that will produce an important benefit for women, then the presumption is that liability is not justified and that the research does not pose great risks to women or their children. In that case, there should be little, if any, need to compensate injuries because there will not be any. On the other hand, if women and children suffer great harm that warrants compensation, then the research must be dangerous. If the research is dangerous, then one must ask whether it is really sufficiently beneficial to justify its being done at all.

A compensation system is sometimes seen as a substitute for tort liability. If people want to avoid liability for injury, they may propose a compensation system to take the place of individual liability. Of course, tort liability is itself one kind of compensation system. So the threshold question is whether any compensation is warranted for particular injuries.

REASONS FOR COMPENSATION

Reasons for compensating injured research subjects tend to fall into three categories: economic, ethical, and political.

Economic Reasons

The economic reason derives from the concept of risk-spreading and the economic theory that the costs of injury should be borne by the person who can best and most efficiently afford them.[1] When injuries occur, there are only two choices: (1) to leave the losses where they lie—with the injured person; or (2) to shift the financial losses to another person—the person who caused the injury, if any, or society as a whole. In most instances, economic theory would favor shifting the losses to a research sponsor or institution[2] because these ordinarily have greater resources than an individual research subject and they can recoup the losses by means of increased prices or other revenue-generating mechanisms. However, given the rarity of research injuries, it is possible that the administrative costs could exceed the efficiency gains of loss shifting.

In practice, economic theory rarely controls policy choices concerning the allocation of losses. Rather, social conceptions of moral rights and duties influence who should bear the financial consequences of different types of injury. This brings us to the second reason for compensating research subjects—ethical principles.

Ethical Reasons

Since the 1960s, individual commentators,[3] and national commissions have agreed that the ethical principles of justice and virtue support, if not require, compensating research subjects who are harmed as a result of participating in research. The ad hoc panel created by the federal government's Department of Health, Education, and Welfare (HEW) to review the Tuskegee Syphilis Study recommended a no-fault compensation system in 1973.[4] The HEW Task Force on the Compensation of Injured Research Subjects recommended compensating injured subjects of research conducted or supported by the Public Health Service in 1977.[5] The National Commission for the Protection of Human Subjects of Biomedical and Behavioral Research, created in 1974, generally endorsed the Task Force's recommendations, but, without studying the issue, recommended only that subjects be told whether or not compensation was available.[6]

In 1982, the President's Commission for the Study of Ethical Problems in Medicine and Biomedical and Behavioral Research found that compensation is appropriate and desirable, but, given the small number of serious injuries arising out of research, could not determine whether there was a need for it.[7] The Commission recommended conducting an experiment to evaluate different compensation systems in pilot settings to see whether their transaction costs and vulnerability to abuse would outweigh their benefits. Unfortunately, no such experiment has been conducted and we have little more information today than the Commission obtained in 1982.

Later in 1982, the World Health Organization and the Council for International Organizations of Medical Sciences issued their Proposed International Guidelines for Biomedical Research Involving Human Subjects based on the World Medical Association's Declaration of Helsinki.[8] The brief Declaration of Helsinki, adopted in 1964, and revised most recently in 1989, has never required compensation for research injuries. The 1982 Proposed Guidelines, however, provided that volunteer subjects are entitled to financial or other assistance to compensate them fully for temporary or permanent disability or death; and endorsed compensation for all research subjects, noting that pharmaceutical manufacturers should assume responsibility for injuries resulting from research they sponsor. A revised version of the Guidelines issued in 1993 states that *every* subject is entitled to equitable compensation.[9] It does make an exception for expected adverse reactions from "investigational therapies or other procedures performed to diagnose or prevent disease." Presumably, this absolves research sponsors of a duty to compensate foreseen adverse reactions in so-called "therapeutic research."

In the United States, no law requires special compensation for research injuries, apart from general tort law principles that apply to everyone. But this could change. In December 1992, for example, Recombinant DNA Advisory Committee of the National Institutes of Health requested the NIH Director to convene a study of how research related nonnegligent injuries should be compensated.[10]

There appear to be three points of view on the issue:

1. That compensation is morally required and not providing it is unjust.

2. That compensation is morally desirable as a charitable act, but not required.

3. That special compensation is not morally required and may even be unjust.

Which point of view one takes depends upon one's conception of research and research subjects. Swazey and Glantz argue that society's conception of its ethical obligation to research subjects may vary depending upon whether subjects are seen as altruistic heros, giftgivers, victims, or willing contractors who assume the risks of research.[11] Heroes volunteer and assume risks for someone else's sake. Since heroes are not supposed to seek any reward, society has no obligation to compensate heroic research subjects. It may *wish* to reward them, however. Similarly, research subjects can be seen as giving a gift to society. Although such donors may not be morally entitled to compensation, society may desire to return the favor by compensating their injuries. Victims appear more entitled to assistance, since the idea of victim connotes someone who has been misused without his consent, such as the Tuskegee Syphilis Study subjects.[12] Victims have a strong moral claim to compensation, especially where society has facilitated the research or benefitted by it. A contractor conjures up the image of a businessman making a bargain, but this suggests that a contractor is entitled to no more than what he or she bargained for, as long as the bargaining process is fair.

These different images lead to two different conceptions of society's obligation. Under the first, which focuses on principles of distributive justice, society has a strong obligation to compensate injured research subjects and not doing so is unjust. Under the second, which focuses on respect for persons and autonomous choices, society has at best a privilege to compensate and not doing so is merely uncharitable, not unjust.

The principle of distributive justice requires that those who take the risks of research should receive the benefits. But the successful product of a research study rarely reaches all the subjects. Compensation is a means of redressing the imbalance between the risks undertaken by research subjects and the benefits that others enjoy as a result. Since most legitimate research is intended to benefit society as a whole, the subject assumes risks for society's sake (some would say making a gift to society). Therefore, society has a moral obligation to make the injured subject whole by compensating those who took the risks and suffered thereby. In addition, it may be argued that where society conducts, supports, or sponsors research, it voluntarily assumes an obligation to compensate those who are injured in its enterprise.

The second conception denies any social obligation to compensate injured research subjects. This view, based on respect for autonomous choices, argues that a research subject who voluntarily participates in research has agreed to assume the risks of research and that providing compensation would be wrong because it does not respect the subject's choice. Insistence on the voluntary consent of the research subject therefore undercuts the subject's claim to compensation. The consent form can be seen as a contract, whereby the subject voluntarily gives up any claim to compensation. Indeed, this is the way in which many consent forms are treated in law.

Women have sometimes pressed their demands to participate in research on the grounds that they are autonomous agents who are morally entitled to make their own decisions about the risks they will assume, especially when they believe they might obtain some benefit thereby. This insistence on autonomy can be turned against women. If the subject assumes the risk, she may forfeit any moral claim to assistance if the risk materializes.

There are two problems with this view, one theoretical, and one empirical. First, it may not be fair to presume that by consenting to participate in research, a subject has assumed the *financial* risks of injury in addition to the physical or medical risks. Moreover, it may be unfair even to ask a subject to assume the financial risks. There are some things, like slavery, that no one is permitted to agree to. The fact that some research may potentially benefit individual subjects does not alter this conclusion. The nature of potential benefits—both to individual subjects and to general knowledge—is relevant to determining whether the research itself is justifiable. But the mere fact that the research is justified because the potential benefits outweigh the potential risks does not dispose of the question whether the subjects must automatically assume the financial consequences of risks they suffer. Potential benefits of research are not a form of compensation for injury.

The empirical problem is that the ideal of perfectly informed, understanding, voluntary consent to participate in research is rarely achieved in practice. Pressure—and sometimes coercion—to participate, the complexity of research, and difficulty in making it understandable work against achieving the ideal. We also do not know whether subjects would consent to waive compensation for injury since they are rarely given the choice. Finally, one can only assume risks of which one has knowledge, so that it seems wrong to presume that anyone would assume financial responsibility for risks that were unknown or unknowable at the time the research began. Although most research consent forms point out that unknown risks are possible, it is unlikely that research subjects really believe that serious injury from unforeseen causes could occur to them.

For these reasons, the view that society has a moral obligation to compensate injured subjects is more persuasive than the view that society has no such duty. Moreover, even if there is no moral duty, society is entitled to choose to provide compensation if it believes it to be beneficial.

Political Reasons

The third category of reasons for providing compensation is political. This is the idea that liability for injuries somehow prevents someone from conducting important research that should be done. A compensation system is frequently proposed to relieve research sponsors of the responsibility for providing compensation, thereby eliminating an obstacle to research. It is thus a policy solution to a possible policy problem. However, the reality of the problem is rarely tested.

Liability for research injuries is a problem only if research organizations are ready, willing, and able to conduct socially beneficial research, *but for* the costs of liability litigation and awards. In the absence of adequate data on liability claims experience from research sponsors, it is impossible to determine whether liability for injuries is a prohibitive financial drain. What few data exist suggest that the current situation differs little from that found by the President's Commission in 1982:[9]

1. The incidence of serious injury and the absolute numbers of people seriously injured are small.

2. Most injuries are trivial in nature and require no medical inter-vention.

3. Of those injuries that require intervention, most are only temporarily disabling.

4. Patient-subjects in therapeutic research are more likely than normal subjects in nontherapeutic research to suffer injury.

In view of the rarity of research injuries, it is pertinent to ask whether there is any need either to limit liability or to assure special compensation to women research subjects. Answering that question requires answering the following two questions: What *might* research sponsors be held responsible for, and what *have* research sponsors been held liable for?

Research sponsors might be held liable for injuries resulting to either women subjects or their later—born children. There appears to be little concern about potential claims by *women* who are injured as a result of participation in research.[13] There is no reason to believe that women are more likely to be injured in research than are men. To the extent that women become a larger proportion of research subjects and make any claims for injury, their claims will merely replace claims that would have been made by men. The small number of such claims suggests that this has not posed a problem for research institutions to date.

Liability for injuries to the children of women research subjects appears to raise fears of substantial financial exposure in some research sponsors.[14] Although tort law has changed over the past 30 years to permit children to sue for some prenatal injuries, the causes of action available to children remain limited.[15,16]

Most involve cases of malpractice by a physician or laboratory actively involved in treating a woman patient, and have no application to research sponsors. Although few drugs have been tested in pregnant women, many drugs have been prescribed for women, both pregnant and not pregnant, and one would expect to find a sampling of adverse reactions to such drugs, perhaps even more than to drugs that had been tested in pregnant women before marketing. However, there are few reported product liability cases alleging injury to a fetus and these are largely confined to intrauterine devices and three drugs:

thalidomide, DES, and bendectin. In some of these cases, like DES, it is hard to argue that there should be no liability. Moreover, these cases involve drugs that were intended to preserve pregnancy and fetal health, so that the fetus can be seen as an intended beneficiary of the drug and a foreseeable victim of injury. The dual concerns about liability and compensation seem to arise out of the idea that people who are injured as a result of research (or anything else, for that matter) deserve compensation, *but* that the sponsors of research should not be responsible for all of the injuries or compensation. This is because many adverse reactions suffered by research subjects are unforeseeable even with the best scientific knowledge and preclinical testing. In such cases, it seems unfair to blame research sponsors for not preventing what they could not reasonably predict. Yet it also seems unfair to leave the entire financial burden (as well as the physical one) on someone who would not have been injured but for participating in the research. In such circumstances, it is reasonable to create a system apart from liability in tort to provide compensation. It also means, however, that research sponsors should only be protected against liability for nonnegligent conduct; they should remain liable for negligent conduct that causes injury. This is because negligence is, by definition, deviation from acceptable standards of conduct. Because negligence is not an intended part of any research, it is not an inherent risk of participating in research. People cannot consent to negligent treatment and research sponsors, like everyone else, remain responsible for injury caused by their own negligence.

TYPES OF COMPENSATION SYSTEMS

There are many ways to provide compensation for research injuries. Choosing among them depends upon the goal sought to be achieved. Following is a summary of the basic policy options (which can be varied to suit specific objectives), what they are designed to accomplish, and their major advantages and disadvantages. They are grouped into three categories: tort liability; mandatory compensation programs; and voluntary or contractual compensation systems.

Tort Liability

Tort law functions, among other things, as one type of compensation system—an indemnity system that makes an individual company or institution responsible for the losses incurred by particular individuals. Historically, it has tied financial responsibility to moral responsibility for injury.[17] More recently, however, liability has also been justified by economic considerations, imposing financial responsibility upon the entity that benefits from an injury-producing enterprise or the entity that can avoid accidents most cheaply.[18]

Limiting liability is not a compensation mechanism, but a cost control measure for research sponsors. Its purpose is to reduce or eliminate financial responsibility for injury in instances in which it is believed that imposing liability on someone is either unjust or unfairly costly. There are three general ways to limit liability for research injuries. The first and broadest is to change tort law to eliminate liability for (nonnegligent) injuries resulting from research. This seems unwarranted in the absence of evidence that research in general gives rise to excessively costly litigation.

If the goal is to reduce the cost of claims from fetuses harmed as a result of research using women subjects, then an alternative would be to change tort law to eliminate specific liability for (nonnegligent) injuries only to such fetuses. Both alternatives guarantee reducing the cost of research, although the absolute amount of savings may be quite small. In both cases, however, it is difficult to justify withdrawing the tort remedy from one class of injured people (those harmed by research) while it is preserved for other classes. (This problem of horizontal justice or equity obtains for most policy options directed at one group.)

A third option is to have the law explicitly recognize that a woman's voluntary, understanding consent to participate in research precludes any claim on behalf of her later-born children that the research harmed them. Where the research is intended to benefit women (as opposed to fetuses or children), there is a good argument that a pregnant woman should be entitled to participate without regard to its effects on the fetus, and that the fetus should not interpose a claim that would discourage the woman from acting in her own best interest. It is also consistent with the idea that women should be free to participate in research regardless of the risk to future children. It is more difficult to ethically justify precluding a cause of action to the fetus, however, where the research is intended to benefit fetuses, as in investigational fetal surgery. As with the first two options, this alternative would probably require state legislation since tort rules are a matter of state law.[19] This raises the practical problem of ensuring consistent laws in all 50 states, the District of Columbia, and the territories. Finally, the major disadvantage of these options is that none offers any assistance to the injured party.

Mandatory Compensation Systems

The term "compensation system" is more often associated with a public program established by state or federal government, such as workers' compensation programs, the federal Black Lung Benefits Act,[20] or the National Vaccine Injury Compensation Program (NVICP).[21] The Federal Employees' Compensation Act (FECA) is the federal equivalent of state workers' compensation programs, and provides compensation for federal civilian employees who are injured in the performance of their employment.[22] It has been extended to apply to other persons who have some connection with the federal government but are not employees, such as Peace Corps and VISTA volunteers and Job Corps participants. The National Institutes of Health has considered the possibility of federal legislation to allow FECA to cover pregnant women research subjects and their later-born children.

Most of these programs offer compensation for injuries resulting from specific causes on a no-fault basis. As long as the injury is demonstrated to result from the specified cause (employment, in the case of workers' compensation; listed vaccines, in the case of the NVICP; and black lung disease in coal miners, in the case of the Black Lung Benefits Act), there is no need to prove negligence or fault in order to recover the available compensation.

No-fault compensation programs offer several advantages over tort litigation. A larger proportion of injuries receive compensation. The costs of administering the system are often less than those of litigation, and a larger percentage of the funds go to the injured parties. There are no "defendants," so parties that might otherwise be liable for injury need not participate in the claims determination process. Finally, the costs are often spread over society, rather than falling randomly on a few institutions. The program can be funded from general tax revenues, as is most appropriate when society as a whole benefits from the activity being protected. Or, where it is important to retain some financial penalty for risk creation, those who create the risks (such as research sponsors) may finance all or part of the system by special taxes.

Compensation programs have disadvantages, however. Any cause-based system raises questions of horizontal justice. As more compensation systems are devised for injuries resulting from particular activities, it becomes more difficult to defend excluding the remaining population of injured people. Those who feel left out may seek to fit their injuries within the definition of compensable harms of special programs. The existence of a compensation program also may attract more claimants than would otherwise seek compensation for their injuries. This may mean that there is a real need for the program. It may mean, however, that people are misattributing accidental injuries to their research experience, and it may raise costs unacceptably high.

Finally, no cause-based system can avoid disputes over the cause of injuries.[23] Determining the cause of injury to a research subject may be even more difficult than finding the cause of other injuries. Most serious research injuries happen to patients who are subjects of therapeutic research, and distinguishing research-related harm from disease-related injury is likely to be especially problematic. Thus, a compensation system for research injuries may offer little savings in time or complexity over litigation.

A fault-based system has the same advantages and disadvantages as a no-fault system, plus an additional disadvantage: the requirement that a claimant prove that someone was negligent or otherwise legally responsible for the injury. In effect, a special compensation system based on fault or negligence, such as the American Medical Association's proposal for malpractice, transfers the litigation process to a more congenial and possibly more efficient and less expensive forum.

It should be remembered that compensation programs only *compensate* injuries *after* they occur. They are not risk prevention or quality assurance mechanisms. If risk prevention is an important goal of research, as it should be, then some other mechanism must be in place to assure that subjects are not placed at any unnecessary risk.

If a compensation system is an appropriate policy option, then the following programmatic issues must be resolved:

Eligibility: Whether to compensate all subjects or only those in "nontherapeutic" research (and whether the therapeutic/nontherapeutic distinction is meaningful for this purpose). Whether to establish geographic or other limits on the characteristics of eligible subjects.

Covered injuries: Whether to provide compensation for all injuries or only for "serious" injuries (however defined) or injuries producing a minimal financial loss. Whether to cover latent injuries arising in the distant future.

Benefits: Whether to reimburse (in addition to medical expenses) actual and estimated losses (e.g., a percentage of individual's wages) or provide a standardized payment (e.g., a percentage of average nonfarm wages) regardless of individual resources. Whether to offer compensation for pain and suffering, and for attorneys' fees incurred.

Payment mechanism: Whether to pay compensation in a lump sum award, in periodic payments, or by means of an annuity (all necessitating estimating future needs) or by means of enrolling the injured party in a medical or disability insurance system.

Administration: What institution should be authorized to make decisions about eligibility for compensation and the amount of awards (e.g., an administrative review board or a court-based procedure).

Review and appeal: Whether claimants should have a right of appeal to the court system or only administrative review of decisions.

Application: Whether the system should have only prospective application or should also apply retrospectively to cover claims of injuries before the effective date.

Ultimately, the fairest compensation system is one that covers all injuries, regardless of cause. This is the only system that avoids the claim of injustice that arises from preferring some injuries over others. It is also likely to be administratively less complex and less expensive than multiple cause-based compensation programs. The more cause-based programs that are advocated, the stronger becomes the case for a universal disability assistance or insurance system. The proposed reform of the health care system promised by the Clinton administration suggests that medical care should become available to all in the future. This should obviate the need for special compensation for medical expenses. It should be noted, however, that the reformed health care system will not necessarily cover injuries resulting from research.

Voluntary and Contractual Systems

Another alternative system for compensating injury is the contract model. The best-known version is that advocated by Professor Jeffrey O'Connell.[24] Applied to research, it would have the research sponsor contractually agree with each research subject, before enrollment, that the sponsor would pay for medical care and some specified losses (usually not including pain and suffering) in the event of a research-related injury. In return, the subject would agree to accept those payments as full compensation and waive any right to sue the sponsor in tort. Ordinarily, there is a time limit in which the sponsor must offer the specified compensation after being notified of a claim.

A contract has the advantage of letting subjects know what they are entitled to before they agree to enroll in a research study, and promises relatively prompt resolution of claims. It has reportedly worked reasonably well in some settings, like school football injuries. However, it is more difficult to predict how it would work with research-related injuries, especially where cause is an issue. Since the sponsor's offer is intended to be less than the complete compensation contemplated by tort law, it might prove less expensive than litigation. However, it is not clear whether research subjects can fully appreciate what they are gaining and giving up when asked to enter into such a contract, and therefore whether it is fair to ask them. While healthy volunteers may feel free to consent or refuse, subjects in therapeutic research may feel pressured to agree to anything.

Some institutions have voluntarily created a compensation system to assist injured research subjects, although not all have told the subjects about them. These may be funded out of the institution's own assets or by commercially purchased insurance. As long as only a few institutions offer such compensation, it may be uneconomic for insurance companies to sell coverage to individual institutions, unless they are very large, since the administrative costs could overwhelm actual payouts. An alternative would be for a group of institutions to create a pooled self-insurance scheme. This would both spread the risk and retain the advantages of self-insurance. Administrative costs should also be minimal.

These voluntary efforts are likely to produce the least expensive compensation system because they substitute an insurance-claims type of procedure for litigation. The disadvantage is that the compensation available is likely to vary from institution to institution, raising questions of horizontal justice.

CONCLUSIONS

If a compensation system is desired, which one is chosen depends upon the goal to be achieved. If the goal is merely to avoid or reduce claims of liability against research sponsors, then the most effective response is not a compensation system at all, but elimination of that liability. This, however, requires a justification for excluding research subjects from a remedy to which everyone else is entitled. If the goal is to compensate all significant injuries resulting from research at the least cost, then the most cost-effective solution would probably be to have research sponsors provide voluntary compensation on a no-fault basis, possibly funded by a self-insurance pool. If the goal is to shift the responsibility for research injuries to society as a whole, regardless of cost, then a federal no-fault compensation program funded by tax revenues (including taxes on research institutions) would serve.

There is really only one reason to adopt a compensation program—recognition of society's ethical obligation to repay those who suffer harm by assuming the risks of socially beneficial research. If society does not feel an ethical obligation to compensate research subjects itself, it may conclude nonetheless that such compensation is the proper responsibility of those who benefit most directly from the research—the sponsors of the research. The cost of compensating injuries can be seen as an ordinary cost of conducting research.

What compensation is *not* is a panacea for fears about liability. Neither is it a guarantee that important research will be done. It would be a mistake to assume that important research to improve women's health will miraculously begin if a compensation program is adopted. Women who are anxious to participate in research should remember that research is not risk free. There are reasons why people worry about research injuries. Our recent experience has been rather positive, with few serious adverse reactions. But history is full of examples of abusing people in the name of research: the Nazi doctors' experiments, the Tuskegee Syphilis Study, the Willowbrook hepatitis B study, to name only a few. The risk of mistreating research subjects by involving them in experiments that should not have been done at all or involving them without their consent is far higher than the risk of injury in a justifiable study. Although the issue of compensating research subjects is important, it is secondary to the question of what research should be done.

NOTES

1. William M. Landes and Richard A. Posner. *The Economic Structure of Tort Law.* Cambridge, Mass.: Harvard University Press, 1987.

2. The phrase "research sponsor" is used as a generic term to include organizations such as pharmaceutical companies that sponsor or conduct research on their own products, public and private institutions such as the National Institutes of Health that fund or conduct research studies and universities and private institutes that carry out research, as well as the individual investigators that perform the research tasks.

3. Irving Ladimer. Clinical Research Insurance. *Journal of Chronic Diseases.* 1963, 16:1229, 1233, Richard P. Bergen. Insurance Coverage for Clinical Investigation. *Journal of the American Medical Association.* 1967, 201:305–306; United States Senate. *Hearings Before the Subcommittee of the Committee on Labor and Public Welfare, Quality of Health Care—Human Experimentation,* Part 3. Statement of Alexander M. Capron, March 7, 1973.

4. Tuskegee Syphilis Study Ad Hoc Advisory Panel. *Final Report.* Washington, D.C.: U.S. Dept. of Health, Education, and Welfare, 1973.

5. Secretary's Task Force on the Compensation of Injured Research Subjects. *Report.* Washington, D.C.: U.S. Dept. of Health, Education, and Welfare, 1977.

6. National Commission for the Protection of Human Subjects of Biomedical and Behavioral Research. *Report and Recommendations: Institutional Review Boards.* Washington, D.C.: U.S. Government Printing Office, 1978.

7. President's Commission for the Study of Ethical Problems in Medicine and Biomedical and Behavioral Research. *Compensating for Research Injuries: The Ethical and Legal Implications of Programs to Redress Injured Subjects,* Vol. 1. Washington, D.C.: U.S. Government Printing Office, 1982.

8. World Health Organization and Council for International Organizations of Medical Sciences. *Proposed International Guidelines for Biomedical Research Involving Human Subjects.* Geneva, Switzerland: CIOMS, 1982.

9. Council for International Organizations of Medical Sciences in collaboration with the World Health Organization. *International Ethical Guidelines for Biomedical Research Involving Human Subjects.* Geneva, Switzerland: WHO, 1993.

10. Rebecca Kolberg. RAC Asks, Who Should Pay for Research Injuries? *Journal of NIH Research.* 1993; 5:37–38.

11. Judith P. Swazey, Leonard Glantz. A Social Perspective on Compensation for Injured Research Subjects. In: President's Commission for the Study of Ethical Problems in Medicine and Biomedical and Behavioral Research. *Compensating for Research Injuries,* Vol. 2, pp. 3–18, 1982.

12. James H. Jones. *Bad Blood: The Tuskegee Syphilis Experiment.* New York, NY: Free Press, 1981.

13. Flannery and Greenberg. Sanford. This volume.

14. L. Elizabeth Bowles. The Disenfranchisement of Fertile Women in Clinical Trials: The Legal Ramifications of and Solutions for Rectifying the Knowledge Gap. *Vanderbilt Law Review.* 1992; 45:877–920.

15. Ellen Wright-Clayton. This volume.

16. See, e.g., Humes v. Clinton, 246 Kan. 590 (1990).

17. Glanville Williams. The Aims of the Law of Tort. *Current Legal Problems.* 1951; 4:137–176.

18. Guido Calabresi. *The Costs of Accidents: A Legal and Economic Analysis.* New Haven, CT: Yale University Press, 1970.

19. *See, e.g.,* McKinstry v. Valley Obstetrics-Gynecology Clinic, 428 Mich. 167 (1987) (Michigan Statute prohibiting minor child from disaffirming arbitration agreements executed by parent on child's behalf held to bind child born after parental consent to arbitration).

20. 30 U.S.C. §§901–945.

21. 42 U.S.C. §§300aa-1 to -34.

22. 5 U.S.C. §§8101 et seq.

23. Wendy K. Mariner. The National Vaccine Injury Compensation Program. *Health Affairs.* 1992; 11:255–265.

24. Jeffrey O'Connell. A "Neo No-Fault" Contract in Lieu of Tort: Preaccident Guarantees of Postaccident Settlement Offers. *California Law Review.* 1985; 73:898–916.

Justice and the Inclusion of Women in Clinical Studies: A Conceptual Framework

Debra A. DeBruin

It often has been charged that women[1] are not adequately included as subjects in clinical research.[2] In particular, it has been charged that women frequently are excluded from studies concerning conditions affecting both women and men, and that when women are included in such studies they tend to be underrepresented.[3]

This Institute of Medicine study of the legal and ethical issues relating to the inclusion of women in clinical studies focusses on this charge of exclusion and underrepresentation. This is a worthy topic for study; the charge demands attention. However, our moral analysis of our practices concerning the inclusion of women in clinical research will fail to capture all that it should if we restrict our focus to the charge of exclusion and underrepresentation.

We must contemplate a more complicated picture. Imagine a society with the following sorts of research practices: women are excluded from and underrepresented in clinical studies concerning conditions affecting both women and men. Even when women are included in adequate numbers in such studies, researchers often fail to do the analysis necessary to determine whether the gender of the study subject affects the results of the study (e.g., whether the condition in question manifests itself differently in women and men; whether the drug on trial affects women and men in different ways). Sometimes when researchers do perform such gender-specific analysis, they do so without regard for advancing knowledge about women's health. (For example, this hypothetical society has a research program that concentrates on the question of how women can pass along certain sexually transmitted diseases to men, but ignores questions of how these diseases affect the women themselves and how they should be treated.) Besides having these practices regarding research into conditions affecting both women and men, our hypothetical society pays relatively little attention to the study of health concerns that are specific to women. In general, then, this hypothetical society fails—not completely, but to a significant extent—to study research questions appropriate for women. It fails, to a significant extent, to include women in its clinical studies—not just in the sense that it fails to include women, or sufficient numbers of women, as subjects, but also in the sense that it fails to incorporate a concern for women's health into its research agenda.

Why should we concern ourselves with this hypothetical society? For one thing, it would be philosophically instructive to develop a moral analysis of this society's research practices. More importantly, however, we should care about this hypothetical society because I have modeled it on our own society. When we realize the society I've described is not really *just* hypothetical, we can begin to see how urgent is the need for moral analysis.

It is difficult to quantify the exact extent of women's exclusion from and underrepresentation in clinical studies in our society. (Indeed, I shall here address only the question of exclusion, since the ambiguity of the term "underrepresentation" makes it so difficult to tell when women are included in "sufficient" numbers and when they are not.[4]) Only since 1992, when the National Institutes of Health revised its policy on the awarding of federal research grants, have researchers been required to include information on gender representation and analysis in their study proposals and renewal requests.[5] Prior to that, information on inclusion was incomplete, and what data there are have not yet been systematically gathered.

Nevertheless, the evidence available so far supports the claim that women have been excluded from clinical studies. The charge of exclusion has been made most conclusively with respect to certain areas of research, e.g., the study of cardiovascular disease. Although cardiovascular disease is the leading cause of death for both women and men, women have been excluded from a number of key studies providing the basis for much of our current understanding of this type of disease—e.g., the Multiple Risk Factor Intervention Trial, conducted on 15,000 men; the Physician's Health Study of aspirin's preventive power against heart disease, conducted on 22,071 men; and "all the large trials on cholesterol-lowering drugs, [which] leave researchers with little or no information about how these drugs work in women."[6]

Some critics of our society's clinical research practices suggest that the exclusion of women is not limited to certain areas of research such as the study of cardiovascular disease, but that it is a systematic problem. These critics note that federal guidelines for research sometimes present barriers to the inclusion of women. For example, until recently, Food and Drug Administration guidelines for drug research advised that women of childbearing potential should be excluded from early phases of drug testing, except in rare cases (e.g., when the inclusion of the women in the drug trial has lifesaving potential for them).[7] Kinney et al. have argued that this policy led, in practice, to the exclusion of women of childbearing potential from later phases of drug testing as well.[8] Moreover, the critics cite suggestive anecdotal evidence to support their claim about the systematic nature of exclusion:

> [T]he first twenty years of a major federal study on health and aging included only men. Yet two-thirds of the elderly population are women. The recent announcement that aspirin can help prevent migraine headaches is based on data from males only, even though women suffer from migraines up to three times as often as men. . . . Most amazing is the pilot project on the impact of obesity on breast and uterine cancer conducted—you guessed it—solely on men. . . . And in basic research, even female rats are frequently excluded as research subjects![9]

We also have evidence that, even when women are included in studies, researchers often fail to perform the analysis that's necessary to determine whether the gender of the research subject affects the results of the study. For example, "there is a premenstrual rise in asthma deaths," but no one has ever studied " 'whether there's a connection between the cycle and the bronchi, or differences in how medications work premenstrually. . . .' "[10] Also, AIDS studies generally fail to include gynecological exams of women subjects, even though AIDS often manifests itself in women through severe, persistent gynecological problems.[11]

When researchers do perform such gender-specific analysis, they sometimes do so without regard for advancing knowledge about women's health. The most shocking example of this phenomenon I'm aware of comes from AIDS research. Most studies of women with AIDS are designed to investigate how women transmit AIDS to their male sex partners or to their fetuses. Faden et al. describe the following study as typical of AIDS research involving women:

> The study, begun in early 1990, is designed to assess whether the rate of HIV transmission from mother to infant can be reduced by continuous oral AZT treatment to HIV-infected pregnant women, intravenous AZT during childbirth, and oral AZT treatment to the newborn infant. The study also seeks to evaluate the safety of AZT for both the pregnant woman and newborn infant. Originally, the study included no maternal health component; attention was focused exclusively on the fetus. No gynecological care was provided to the women, there was no requirement that an internist be included on the study team to meet the women's non-obstetrical health needs, and AZT for the women was discontinued immediately after delivery. . . . The Women's Health Core Committee of the [AIDS Clinical Trial Group] revised the protocol in 1991. Under the changed protocol, whatever treatment the women had been receiving during the study

would be continued for six weeks postpartum, while the infants would continue to receive their study treatment for eighteen months.[12]

Faden et al. also note that "[g]iven that the first cases of AIDS in women were reported to the CDC in 1981 and the number of AIDS cases has been rising faster in women than in men nearly every year since 1986, it is extraordinary that the NIH's first major study of how HIV disease manifests itself and progresses in women will not begin accruing patients before the end of 1994."[13]

Finally, critics commonly charge that health concerns that are specific to women receive relatively little research attention. The long list of oft-cited gaps in women's health research includes study of "the effects of hormone replacement therapy in reducing heart disease and bone loss, the impact of a low-fat diet on preventing breast cancer, and the use of vitamin D and calcium supplements to prevent bone loss and reduce colon cancer."[14]

In this paper, then, I shall assume that (1) women are excluded from and underrepresented in clinical studies; (2) even when women are included in sufficient numbers, researchers often fail to perform the analysis necessary to determine whether the gender of the research subject affects the results of the study; (3) when researchers do perform gender-specific analysis, they sometimes do so without regard for advancing knowledge about the health of women; and (4) health concerns specific to women receive little research attention. I shall not—I cannot—make any definitive empirical claims about the full extent of these phenomena. However, I shall say this: We must not so focus on any individual phenomenon that we lose sight of the complete picture composed of all four phenomena. Given this complete picture, I shall reiterate that our society fails—not completely, but to a significant extent—to study research questions appropriate for women. It fails, to a significant extent, to include women in its clinical studies—not just in the sense that it fails to include women, or sufficient numbers of women, as subjects, but also in the sense that it fails to incorporate a concern for women's health into its research agenda. Whatever the extent of this failure, I shall argue that it is morally unacceptable wherever it occurs. I shall argue that these research practices result from and further perpetuate the oppression of women in our society. (Toward this end, I shall present an analysis of some aspects of women's oppression.) Given this connection between the oppression of women and these research practices, and given the systematic nature of oppression, it would be quite surprising if this failure to incorporate a concern for women's health into the research agenda were limited to isolated areas of research.

I shall also assume that these practices concerning the inclusion of women in clinical studies result in inequalities in the quality and availability of care, which have a detrimental impact on women's health. After a two-year study, the Public Health Service Task Force on Women's Health Issues concluded in its 1985 report that "[t]he historical lack of research focus on women's health concerns has compromised the quality of health information available to women as well as the health care they receive."[15] It stands to reason that this is true for health concerns specific to women. When these concerns are not studied, but those specific to men are, there will be inequalities in the availability and quality of care. When women cannot get care for their conditions because those conditions haven't been studied, or when they get care based on inadequate information about their conditions, their health will inevitably suffer. Further, there is evidence that this assumption is true for conditions that affect both men and women. For example, there is evidence that, because of the way women have been included in (or to a large extent excluded from) AIDS research, women with AIDS receive less, and lower quality, care than their male counterparts. There is also evidence that some drugs interact with women's menstrual cycles so that drug regimens based on studies that that excluded women or failed to perform gender-specific analysis are ineffective or harmful for women. There is much we don't know about how women's health is affected by our practices concerning their inclusion in studies, precisely because the relevant studies have not been done. What we do know gives us cause for worry.[16]

My aim in this paper is to provide a framework for thinking about two broad philosophical questions: (1) Are our practices concerning the inclusion of women in clinical studies unjust, and, if so, why? And (2) if they are unjust, what sorts of remedies ought we to adopt?

THE INJUSTICE OF OUR PRACTICES

Are our practices concerning the inclusion of women in clinical studies unjust? The answer, in a word, is yes. I shall devote this section to an analysis of *why* they are unjust.

To answer this question, we need some understanding of what justice requires. Contemporary philosophers typically embrace what I'll call "the distributive paradigm of justice."[17] That is, they typically define justice as the proper distribution of benefits and burdens among individuals in a society. Then, as one would imagine, they disagree about what makes such a distribution "proper."

In her recent book, *Justice and the Politics of Difference*, Iris Marion Young argues that the distributive paradigm of justice fails to capture all there is to justice. In the first place, she contends, not all of the concerns of justice are matters of the distribution of benefits and burdens. Oppression qualifies as a concern of justice—indeed, justice requires that we eliminate oppression—but some important aspects of oppression are not purely matters of distribution. (I'll talk more about this later.) In the second place, Young notes, the distributive paradigm considers only how social arrangements affect individuals as such. She argues that such an exclusive focus on individuals fails to capture important aspects of justice. After all, people are oppressed not as individuals, but as members of groups. Therefore, Young concludes, we need a broader characterization of justice than the distributive paradigm provides, one that recognizes both distributive and nondistributive matters as concerns of justice and acknowledges the moral significance of both individuals and social groups.

I agree with Young about these matters, and so I propose that we accept the broader characterization of justice. Of course, this does not provide us with anything approaching a complete account of what justice requires. Still, it gives us enough of a basis for discussion so that we can achieve a reasonable understanding of the issues confronting us.

I suggest that we focus on particular considerations that might be offered in arguing for or against our practices concerning the inclusion of women in clinical studies and see why we must conclude, all things considered, that they are unjust. Let's begin by discussing considerations weighing against our practices concerning the inclusion of women. First, we must take into account the detrimental effects we're assuming these practices will have on women's health: the deaths, the disabilities, the illnesses, the suffering.[18] Second, we must note how these negative health effects can result in further disadvantages to women, such as time lost from work and impaired ability to function in personal relationships. Third, we must see that these harms to women can negatively affect those who have relationships with the women who suffer—their employers or employees, their friends and lovers, their children. Even purely distributive models of justice would have to take all these concerns into account. And these concerns alone weigh heavily against our practices concerning the inclusion of women in clinical studies.

But the distributive considerations are compounded by nondistributive ones. We must recognize that it's no accident that women suffer the harms I've just listed. Rather, these harms are one result of the oppression of women in our society, and, accordingly, they become a part of that oppression. How are these harms the result of oppression? There's a lot one could say about this, but I would like to focus on how two particular aspects of oppression can give rise to these harms.

One central aspect of oppression concerns how groups, and individuals in those groups, are conceived of in society. Let me explain. Oppressive societies take the dominant group's identity and experience to be, not the particular identity or experience of one group in society, but the universal identity and experience—that is, the norm.[19] I shall call this aspect of oppression "false universalism." The upshot for our discussion here is this: Our society does not conceive of men in terms of their gender; it conceives of them gender-neutrally, as persons. Thus, men's identity and experience serves, in effect, as the characterization or standard of what it is to be a person. This is true only of men's identity and experience; it is not true of women's.

According to sociologists Kimmel and Messner, there is a sociological explanation for this conceptual phenomenon. "[T]he mechanisms that afford us privilege are very often invisible to us. . . . Thus, white people rarely think of themselves as 'raced' people, rarely think of race as a central element in their experience."[20] (Hence we use the phrase "people of color" to refer to everyone but white people.) According to Kimmel and Messner, the same point holds for gender. That is, men rarely think of themselves as gendered persons, rarely think of gender as a central element in their experience. Indeed, Kimmel and Messner suggest that white men, when asked what kind of being they see when they look at themselves in the mirror, tend to respond "a person" or "a human" (race- and gender-neutral), but white women tend to respond "a woman" (race-neutral but gender-specific), and black women tend to respond "a black woman" (race- and gender-specific).[21]

Our use of language further bears out the point that our society takes men's identity and experience as the characterization or standard of what it is to be a person. After all, the way we talk reflects the way we think. In our language, masculine terms such as "he" and "man" serve as gender-neutral terms; feminine terms such as "she" and "woman" cannot.[22] Also, we qualify gender-neutral occupation names when women, but not when men, hold the occupation in question. For example, we speak of "women doctors," "women professors," and "lady cops" but not "male doctors," "men professors," or "gentleman cops." Her gender is relevant; his is not. She is conceived of in gendered terms; he is not. His identity and experience serves as the characterization or standard of what it is to be a doctor, professor, police officer—or even a person.

False universalism has two consequences. First, it makes women invisible in the following sense. When we think "person," we tend to think not of women but of our paradigm persons—men. Women tend to disappear from the conceptual scene when we're thinking in gender-neutral terms, because we tend to think of women in terms of their gender. On the other hand, men tend not to disappear, because we tend not to conceive of men in gender-specific terms but as the standard of what it is to be a person. The second consequence of false universalism is that, insofar as they are different from men, women are conceived of as inferior, deficient, or deviant. If they were not, if their differences were viewed as *mere* differences, this would challenge men's claim to universality, their ability to serve as the standard of what it is to be a person.

We should note that while false universalism qualifies as a concern of justice, it is not purely a matter of the distribution of benefits and burdens among individuals in society. Rather, this aspect of oppression is primarily a matter of our conceiving of men in gender-neutral terms, as the norm of personhood, and of women in gendered terms, as deviant from this norm. More generally, then, false universalism is primarily a matter of how we conceive of women and men in our society. How we conceive of men and women does have some distributive consequences, e.g., the allocation of resources for studies of men's or women's health concerns, but how we conceive of men and women cannot be satisfactorily analyzed as a matter of the distribution of benefits and burdens. Thus, a purely distributive model of justice could not fully account for this concern of justice; to do so, we need the sort of broader model Young provides.

A *second* important aspect of oppression is that society subordinates members of oppressed groups to members of dominant groups.[23] Domination and subordination are typically analyzed as imbalances of power. However, this is too simplistic an account of dominance and subordination.

In the first place, such an account fails to recognize the source of whatever power imbalances are involved in dominance and subordination. These power imbalances arise from socially prescribed norms. Let me explain. Society establishes norms that apply to individuals on the basis of their membership in certain groups. What these social norms do is prescribe what members of particular groups should be like. Thus, these norms fix (parts of) our social conceptions of members of particular groups. For example, gender norms prescribe what roles and responsibilities women should assume, how women should look, walk, talk, sit, interact with others, and much more. In general, they provide us with a picture of what a "real" or a "good" woman is like. That is, gender norms specify how we are to conceive of men and women in our society.[24] Moreover, the social reality of who gets how much and what kinds of power is built into these social conceptions of groups. Perhaps the most obvious example of this connection between power and norms is this: In many societies, "good" women are not aggressive or ambitious, though "good" men are. These gender norms condemn women, but praise men, for possessing traits that in many ways give individuals power. Therefore, any analysis of the social reality about power relations must be given in terms of the social conception of groups.

Further, it is a mistake to think that all dominance and subordination is a matter of imbalances of power. Sometimes—indeed, probably far more often than not—women's subordination to men is a matter of women's interests being taken less seriously than are men's, or of the arenas in which women have power (indeed, more power than men have) being valued less than those in which men have power. For example, in our society, women have primary responsibility for domestic concerns; thus, in day-to-day matters, women often have more power in the domestic sphere than men do. (Indeed, women often almost single-handedly run the home.) Men, on the other hand, (still) have more power than women in the world of paid employment and in politics. But work and power in the public sphere (paid employment, politics) are highly valued in our society, whereas work and power in the domestic sphere are not.

We should note that, on the standard account of dominance and subordination, it appears that we can analyze this aspect of oppression on a purely distributive model of justice. Assuming we can speak meaningfully of the distribution of abstract goods like power,[25] the standard account says simply that society allocates power (or certain kinds or amounts of power) to members of some groups but not to others. I have just argued that this account of dominance and subordination is overly simplistic. On the more realistic account I have just sketched, dominance and subordination cannot be analyzed in purely distributive terms. There are two reasons for this. First, on my account, dominance and subordination is sometimes a matter of power imbalances. However, I have argued that the social reality of who gets how much and what kinds of power is built into the social conceptions of groups provided by our social norms. Since, as we have seen, we cannot give a purely—even a primarily—distributive account of our social conceptions of groups, and since an analysis of domination and subordination must be given in terms of an account of our social conception of groups, we cannot give a purely—even a primarily—distributive account of dominance and subordination. Second, on my account, sometimes dominance and subordination is not a matter of imbalances of power, but instead a matter of women's interests being taken less seriously than men's are, or of the arenas in which women have power (indeed, more power than men have) being valued less than those in which men have power. These aspects of dominance and subordination cannot satisfactorily be analyzed in terms of the distribution of benefits and burdens to individuals in society. For these two reasons, purely distributive models of justice could not fully account for domination and subordination, even though it is a concern of justice. To fully account for dominance and subordination, we need the sort of broader model Young provides.

Now what does all this discussion of oppression have to do with the harms we've decided women suffer as a result of our practices concerning their inclusion in clinical studies? Lots. Remember that my claim is that women suffer these harms because given our practices, we fail to incorporate a concern for women's health into our research agenda, and that we fail to do so because of women's oppressed place in our society. I'd like to suggest three links between women's oppression and our practices concerning their inclusion in clinical studies. First, we've seen that oppression makes women invisible. Acknowledging this allows us to come to an important realization: we can abhor oppression without necessarily vilifying men. In the case at hand, we need not assume that members of the medical establishment sit around consciously thinking, "We're men, and we have the power to determine what will be studied and what will not. We will promote research on men's health issues, and, for the most part, ignore women's health issues." Instead, we can see how the oppression of women creates in men a conceptual blindness to the special needs of women.

Second, we've seen that oppression makes women appear deviant or problematic. We know that one of the reasons that women have traditionally been excluded from clinical studies of conditions that affect both men and women is that, as *The Washington Post* put it, "their hormonal fluctuations [have been] said to 'confound' or confuse research results."[26] Women's cycles appear not only to be different from men's physiology, but also to be problematic. Because men are conceived of in gender-neutral terms as paradigmatic persons, researchers too often feel they can simply avoid the "problems" caused by women's cycles by studying only men. (I'll have more to say about this below.)

Third, we've seen that oppression imposes gender norms on women which subordinate women to men. These gender norms can dictate what research will be done and what will not.[27] For example, consider research on birth control methods. By far most of this research focuses on birth control methods for women. In our society, social norms place primary responsibility for birth control on women; this norm is usually understood as developing out of the norms that give women primary responsibility for children. These norms contribute to women's subordinate status in society by demanding that women devote themselves to child care—undervalued labor in our society—while men are freed to advance their status in more highly valued activities, and to pursue leisure activities. The birth control research agenda based on these norms also subordinates women's interests to men's. Women must bear the costs of birth control: the inconvenience of acquiring it, which often requires a visit to her doctor for a prescription; the monetary cost of purchasing it; the psychological costs of bearing responsibility for its proper use, which are not inconsiderable especially since our gender norms frown on women who plan for sex; the physical costs of using it, from discomfort to serious health risks. Men needn't bear these costs, but they do reap the benefits of women's sacrifices.

Consider another example of how gender norms can influence research agendas. In our society women's primary sex roles are those of wife and mother. These roles define women in terms of their relations to men and children, they require that women provide service to their men and children, and they take priority over the woman's other roles—e.g., of career person, or of caretaker for herself. Thus, these roles subordinate women to others. Society's conception of women in terms of their relations to men and children influences research agendas. For example, we've seen that as far as AIDS research goes, women have been primarily studied as "vectors" of the disease. That is, research on women concentrates on how women transmit AIDS to their male sex partners and their children. In contrast, little research has been done on how AIDS affects women themselves.[28] Here women's interests are subordinated to those of their men and children.

Thus we can see that our practices concerning the inclusion of women in studies and the harms attendant upon these practices are one result of the oppression of women in our society, and, accordingly, they become a part of that oppression. Since justice requires the elimination of oppression, this serves as an especially powerful consideration weighing against our practices concerning the inclusion of women in clinical studies. Notice that this consideration would weigh against our practices even if they did not have a detrimental impact on women's health. Insofar as these practices result from and are a part of women's oppression, they must be remedied out of a moral concern for the elimination of oppression, no matter what additional harms are related to the practices.

What considerations purport to weigh in favor of our practices concerning the inclusion of women in clinical studies? I shall focus on three such types of considerations. First, we must take into account the role played by considerations of cost in attempts to justify these practices. There's no doubt that including women in sufficient numbers and doing gender-specific analysis would increase the costs of studies. There's no doubt that limits in our resources force us to face difficult decisions about how to allocate those resources. However, it is morally unacceptable to allocate resources on the basis of sex (or, for that matter, other group membership, such as race, sexual preference, etc.) when there is so much at stake for the excluded parties. It would be outrageously immoral to manage the costs of education by excluding, say, black children from our educational system. Likewise, we must conclude that considerations of cost cannot justify failing to include women in clinical studies in sufficient numbers or failing to perform gender-specific analysis.

Second, as we've seen, researchers often try to justify excluding women from studies of conditions that affect both men and women by appealing to the claim that women's hormonal fluctuations "'confound' or confuse research results." However, as we've also seen, this purported justification takes women's cycles not only to be different from men's physiology, but also to be problematic. Hence this purported justification must be rejected because of its connection to the first aspect of oppression I discussed above—false universalism. Moreover, it would be appropriate to strive for clean, uniform data which can be analyzed using simple, elegant models only if such research best served the health care needs of all persons. But we know that it does not, since we know that some diseases present themselves differently in women than in men, and that some treatments affect women differently than men. Therefore, we have ample reason to reject this purported justification.

Third, it is sometimes argued that we should exclude women of childbearing age from clinical studies to protect the well-being of possible or actual fetuses. A full discussion of this issue would require a paper—or a book—of its own. Here I shall briefly make five points: (1) It is not morally acceptable to place a higher value on fetal life and well-being than on women's lives and well-being. If we refuse to study women of childbearing age because we are concerned for the well-being of (possible or actual) fetuses, regardless of the health benefits to women such research would yield, then we place a higher value on fetal life and well-being than on women's lives and well-being. Current regulations require researchers to consider the impact of research only on individual women actually involved in the research and on (actual or possible) fetuses affected by the research. In the cases of both actually pregnant women and women of childbearing potential who are not pregnant, regulations deny (or, in the case of nonpregnant women, have until recently denied) women participation in studies unless the purpose of the research is to meet the significant health needs of the individual women in the study.[29] The impact research would have on the health of women as a group (not just those involved in the study) is ignored. If we omit from our risk-benefit analysis, or refuse to weigh, the possible benefits the research would have for women's health generally, then we fail to place sufficient value on the health of women in general[30]—we value fetal life and well-being more highly than women's lives and well-being. We cannot be morally justified in doing so. (2) Assuming that we have a legitimate moral interest (at least in some cases) in protecting fetal well-being, we should strive to find a way to safeguard (possible or actual) fetuses while conducting research on women. We should not simply settle for excluding women from research. (3) No matter what view we take about the value of fetal life and well-being, this consideration cannot justify excluding from clinical studies women who cannot or will not have children.[31]   (4) If we are concerned with fetal life and well-being, then we must take care not only with how we conduct research on women, but also with how we conduct research on men. We have reason to believe that fetal health and well-being is affected not only by agents to which women are exposed, but also by those to which men are exposed. To exclude women but not men from research out a concern for fetal health (as current regulations do) is to discriminate unjustly against women.[32] (5) Comments (1)–(4) discuss moral considerations involved in the exclusion of women from research out of a concern with fetal health. Some researchers wish to exclude women not so much out of a moral concern for the health of the fetus, but out of a concern for avoiding legal liability for the possible harms fetuses might suffer as a result of research. I cannot discuss liability laws at any length here. I shall say only that our liability laws should be consistent with our moral views on this matter.

It should be clear by now why our practices concerning the inclusion of women in clinical studies are unjust. We now understand the considerations arguing for and against these practices, and there can be no doubt that the considerations against these practices vastly outweigh those supporting them.

REMEDIES

Now that we have a reasonable understanding of why our practices concerning the inclusion of women are unjust, we can turn our attention to what we should do to remedy this injustice. It should be clear by now that we must do *something*; justice cannot tolerate the preservation of the status quo. Where these injustices occur, they must be remedied. The question is: What kind of new policy should we adopt? Of course, any policy we adopt must require more than mere head counting. That is, simply adding more women to studies will not solve the injustices in question here. We must explore whether the sex of the subject is relevant to the condition or treatment being studied. We must not treat women's bodies as deviant or problematic compared to men's when we do so, nor should we treat our study of women as a mere means to gaining knowledge of the health of men and children. However, it is not enough for us to realize how we should proceed once we've included women in our studies. We must also determine how we should allocate the resources available to support research. It is this question that I shall focus on in this section of this paper.

Should we demand gender-neutral allocation of resources for research? In general, gender-neutral policies require us to ignore gender when we reason from the point of view of justice, and prohibit us from treating persons differently on the basis of their gender. Thus, such a policy would require nondiscrimination in the allocation of resources for research. With respect to studies of conditions affecting both men and women, it would require that women be included in studies in sufficient numbers. To exclude or underrepresent women would be to extend special treatment to men—i.e., desirable levels of inclusion in studies—which we would deny to women. With respect to studies of health concerns specific to women, a gender-neutral policy would require that resources for research be allocated on the basis of the same criteria we use to allocate resources for studies of men's health—e.g., how many people are affected by it, how much of a health threat it is.

Or should we insist upon something more than gender-neutrality? Should we adopt (at least temporarily) programs of preferential treatment which allocate a larger share of available resources to studies of women's health than would be allocated by a gender-neutral policy? I shall argue that we should, indeed, adopt a policy of preferential treatment as a remedy for the injustices involved in our practices concerning the inclusion of women in clinical studies. I shall begin by dispensing with the main argument against preferential treatment.

The most common argument against preferential treatment goes like this: "Programs involving preferential treatment discriminate in favor of members of certain groups. But all discrimination is unjust. Therefore, programs involving preferential treatment are unjust." We must reject this argument, since it depends upon an ambiguity in the meaning of the term "discrimination."

"Discrimination" can mean simply "the drawing of a distinction" or it can mean "the unjust drawing of a distinction." When the opponent of preferential treatment claims, in the first step of the argument, that such treatment discriminates, she cannot mean that it discriminates unjustly. That would be to assume what the argument was supposed to demonstrate. So, at this point in the argument, to say that preferential treatment discriminates is just to say that it draws distinctions. That, of course, is true. But in that case the next step in the argument—the claim that all discrimination is unjust—is false. Not all distinction drawing is unjust. The claim that all discrimination is unjust turns out to be true only if, at this point in the argument, "discrimination" means "the unjust drawing of a distinction." But logic prohibits changing the meaning of key terms from one step in an argument to another. So either the argument assumes what it is supposed to establish, or it contains false assumptions, or it contains a prohibited shift in the meaning of a key term. Thus, we must reject the argument.

So we have no reason to believe that programs of preferential treatment are inherently unjust. But what reason do we have to believe that we would be justified in adopting such a program as a remedy for the injustices involved in our practices concerning the inclusion of women in clinical studies? I shall argue that we have plenty of reason to believe that we would be justified in adopting such a program. Indeed, I shall argue that justice not only permits but *requires* that we adopt such a program. Let's begin by considering what justice requires of a remedy for the injustices involved in the way we've included women in clinical studies.

Most generally, of course, a remedy must correct the injustices in question. In this case, this means it must address both the distributive and the nondistributive injustices. Because we traditionally have conceived of justice on the distributive paradigm, we are accustomed to focusing only on distributive injustices. But we must not lose sight of the nondistributive ones. Even if it were to turn out, contrary to all evidence and reasonable expectations, that our practices concerning the inclusion of women in clinical studies have had no detrimental impact on women's health whatsoever, we would still have to remedy serious, albeit nondistributive, injustices. For example, we would still have to counter the injustices involved in the way we conceive of women in our society, as reflected in our medical research. Even if all the data that we gather from men apply perfectly well to women, it still says something disturbing about how we conceive of men and women in this society if we continue to study only men: it says that men are the norm for persons, and that, when we're thinking in gender-neutral terms of persons, we needn't think of (or include) women.

In addition, a remedy must respond to a cross-temporal perspective on the moral problems in question.[33] That is, the remedy must address the important realization that our practices concerning the inclusion of women in studies have created justice problems in the past, continue to create such problems in the present (both because their use in the past has deprived us of knowledge crucial to the treatment of women now, and because the practices continue in the present), and will continue to create justice problems in the future unless something is done to solve all these problems.

I contend that a gender-neutral policy cannot correct the injustices involved in our practices concerning the inclusion of women in clinical studies. I shall outline three reasons why such a policy cannot correct those injustices.

The first two reasons concern the inability of the gender-neutral policy to respond to a cross-temporal perspective on the injustices in question. *First, such a gender-neutral policy cannot correct for past or present injustices; it is completely future-oriented.* When we confront the problem of our failure to incorporate a concern for women's health into our research agenda, we face a history of injustice (involving, as we have seen, both distributive and nondistributive injustices). A gender-neutral policy of nondiscrimination says, in effect, "We'll try to do better in the future, by resolving to incorporate a concern for women then." But simply resolving to do better in the future does nothing to address past or present injustices. True, we cannot resolve to do better in the future without acknowledging past or present injustices. But to acknowledge past or present injustices is not to make amends for them. And we must make amends; justice requires it. Suppose, for example, that there is a society that has a history of the following practice: white people (the dominant race by this society's standards) routinely steal the property of black people. Suppose further that this society sanctions, or at least does not condemn, this practice. Suppose finally that members of this society come to be persuaded that this practice is unjust, and that they decide to remedy the injustice by resolving not to allow whites to steal the property of blacks in the future. This example makes it clear that, when we are faced with a history of injustice, simply stopping the unjust practice, while important, is not sufficient from the point of view of justice. Justice requires that amends be made for past and present injustices. In our hypothetical example, justice requires, for example, that restitution be made to those who have had their property taken from them unjustly. A gender-neutral policy of nondiscrimination simply stops our problematic practices concerning the inclusion of women in clinical studies. Thus, it makes no provision for making amends for past or present injustices. Therefore, a gender-neutral policy of nondiscrimination does not correct for past or present injustices, and so it does not meet the demands of justice.

Opponents of preferential treatment sometimes argue that, while it makes sense to think that we're obligated to compensate individuals we have wronged, it makes no sense to think we're obligated to compensate certain individuals now for wrongs done by others to others in the past. While this objection may seem initially plausible, it cannot succeed in undermining my claim that justice requires us to make amends for past and present injustices, for two reasons:

(1) This objection cannot undercut my claim that we must make amends for present injustices; it addresses only past injustices (and, indeed, only those injustices done so far in the past that neither those who perpetrated them or benefitted from them nor those who suffered them are alive any longer).

(2) This objection cannot subvert my claim that we must make amends for past injustices, for three reasons: (a) It fails to recognize that those past injustices, done by others against others (if committed far enough in the past) have present unjust consequences—for example, women now suffer from lack of appropriate health care as a result of our practices concerning the inclusion of women in studies in the past. (b) The objection equates *making amends* for past injustices with *paying compensation* for past injustices. But paying compensation is merely one way of making amends. This is a point that never seems to be recognized in discussions of affirmative action and preferential treatment. Consider the following case: Dr. Jones commits malpractice, and Samantha Smith dies as a result. Jones can justly be required to compensate the Smith family for the loss of Samantha's earnings. He cannot, however, justly be required to compensate the Smith family for the loss of Samantha. It is morally inappropriate to speak in terms of paying compensation here, because one cannot put a price on human life which one can then pay in exchange for taking the life. It is not at all inappropriate, however—indeed, quite the contrary—to talk of Dr. Jones making amends for his actions which led to Samantha's death. So even if, as the objection alleges, we ought not require certain individuals to pay compensation to other individuals now for injustices performed by others against others in the past (and even this is false, I think), it does not follow that we ought not require certain individuals to make amends to other individuals now for injustices performed by others against others in the past. (c) The objection loses sight of the moral importance of groups; it focuses solely on compensation (or, if we revise it in light of my previous point, making amends) to specific individuals who have suffered injustices. However, the broader conception of justice I have adopted in this paper opens up the possibility of thinking in terms of making amends to groups, not just to individuals. After all, individual women suffer the injustices involved in our research practices not because they are the individuals they are but because they are women. Furthermore, *all* women (just because they are women) risk the harms to health and other related harms I listed early on in my analysis of why these practices are unjust. And *all* women, just because they are women, suffer in some way from the oppression of women in our society (especially the aspects of oppression concerning how we conceive of women). Thus it makes perfect sense to speak of society making amends to women (as a group) for the injustices it has perpetrated against women (as a group).

The second reason why a gender-neutral policy cannot correct the injustices involved in our research practices is that such a policy, although it is completely future-oriented, cannot fully correct for future injustices. As I argued above, such a policy does serve as a resolution to incorporate a concern for the health of women into our research agenda in the future. And that is, admittedly, an important part of correcting for the future injustices in question. But it is not all there is to it. Even if we were to incorporate a concern for women's health into our research agenda immediately, our history of failing to do so would continue to affect people in this society for a long, long time to come. For example, men would continue to receive better health care than they would have received in a truly just society, because a disproportionate share of our resources have for so long gone to the study of men's health. On the other hand, women would continue to be the victims of these inequalities in the availability and quality of care. Adopting a gender neutral policy of nondiscrimination might well stop those inequalities from broadening, but it would do nothing to narrow them. Justice requires that we close those gaps; since these inequalities are unjust, allowing them to continue is unjust. Since a gender-neutral policy of nondiscrimination would allow them to continue, it cannot correct for all the future injustices involved in our history of failing to incorporate a concern for women's health into our research agenda.

The third reason why a gender-neutral policy cannot correct for the injustices involved in our practices concerning the inclusion of women in clinical studies is that gender-neutrality provides an unacceptable model of what constitutes justice. Gender-neutral policies are premised on the idea that a person's gender is irrelevant from the point of view of justice. That is, they are based on the view that all persons should be treated equally, regardless of their gender. Thus, they require us to ignore gender when we reason from the point of view of justice, and they prohibit us from treating persons differently on the basis of their gender. Such a model of justice fails to incorporate a sufficient and appropriate moral sensitivity to our social context. We live in a society with a history of gender-based oppression. Gender-neutral models do condemn oppression as they understand it; they contend that it is unjust for women to be treated differently from men on the basis of their gender. However, such models of justice do not recognize that *our history of gender-based oppression makes gender relevant from the point of view of justice.*[34]

A concern with justice demands that we strive to recognize, to understand, and to overcome oppression. So, as we have seen, we must concern ourselves with (among other things) the intricacies of our oppressive social conception of women, and with the multifarious ways this social conception has affected, and continues to affect, women. We must resist and revise our oppressive conception of women. We must make amends for our history of oppression. We must eliminate gender-based inequalities that oppression has created. To accomplish all of this, we must attend to gender when we reason from the point of view of justice. None of this is compatible with a model of justice that requires us to ignore gender in our justice reasoning and prohibits us from treating persons differently on the basis of their gender. For example, we could not make amends to women for our history of oppressing them (with all the complex varieties of injustices that involves) if we did not attend to gender in our justice reasoning and extend special treatment to women that we denied to men; quite simply, in our society, women are in a position that calls for the making of amends, and men, as such, are not.[35] Also, we could not eliminate existing gender-based inequalities if we did not attend to gender in our justice reasoning and extend special treatment to women that we denied to men; again, in our society, women are in a social position that calls for their being advanced to a point of equity with men, and men, as such, are not in such a position vis-a-vis women. In general, since we live in a society with a history of gender-based oppression, adopting a stance of gender-neutrality blinds us to—forces us to ignore—issues that are relevant from the point of view of justice, and prohibits us from correcting the injustices of oppression since doing so necessitates that we extend special treatment to women which we deny to men.[36]

We have seen that there are three reasons why a gender neutral policy of nondiscrimination cannot meet the demands of justice: (1) it cannot correct for past and present injustices; (2) it cannot correct for future injustices; and (3) given the context of our oppressive society, gender-neutrality provides an unacceptable model of what constitutes justice. For all these reasons, we must reject such gender-neutral policies as remedies for the injustices involved in the exclusion of women from clinical studies.

Programs of preferential treatment, on the other hand, can meet the demands of justice. Recall that, most generally, justice demands that a remedy correct the injustices in question. More specifically, justice first requires that a remedy address both the distributive and the nondistributive injustices involved in our practices concerning the inclusion of women in clinical studies. I have argued that, even if these practices had no detrimental impact on women's health, justice would still require us to adopt a remedy that could counter the nondistributive injustices involved in our practices: the way we conceive of women, and the subordinate weight we give to their interests or value we attach to the arenas in which they have power, as these things are reflected in our medical research. A policy of preferential treatment would counter these injustices in two ways. First, by requiring us to incorporate a concern for women's health into our research agenda, it would help undermine the subordination of women and the false universalist view that men are the norm for persons and that, when we're thinking in gender-neutral terms of persons, we needn't think of (or include) women. Second, by requiring us to extend special treatment to women, it would not merely reject these aspects of women's oppression, it would also make amends for our history of oppression (something a gender-neutral policy could not do).

Second, justice requires that a remedy respond to a cross-temporal perspective on the moral problems in question. I have argued that gender-neutral policies fail to meet this demand of justice. Unlike such policies, policies of preferential treatment can meet this demand. Unlike gender-neutral policies, policies of preferential treatment can make amends for past and present injustices by offering special treatment to women—that is, by not only resolving to incorporate a concern for women's health into our research agenda in the future, but also going the extra distance to make up for the various (distributive and nondistributive) injustices of the past and present. Also, unlike gender-neutral policies, policies of preferential treatment can fully correct for future injustices. That is, not only can it halt our problematic practices concerning the inclusion of women in studies, but by allocating extra resources to the study of women's health, it can work to close the gaps between men's and women's health care, to eliminate the inequalities in quality and availability of care that our history of these problematic practices has created.

Finally, I have argued that gender neutral policies fail to meet the demands of justice because gender-neutrality provides an unacceptable model of what constitutes justice. Unlike such policies, programs of preferential treatment recognize that our history of gender-based oppression makes gender relevant from the point of view of justice. Unlike gender neutral policies, programs of preferential treatment allow—even require—us to take gender into account when we reason from the point of view of justice, and permit—even require—us to extend special treatment to women that we deny to men. As I have just shown, this insures that such programs can make amends for past and present injustices and can eliminate existing inequalities between men's and women's health care, as justice requires a remedy to do.

In summary, then, gender-neutral policies fail to meet the demands of justice, while policies of preferential treatment succeed in doing so. Therefore, justice requires that we adopt a policy of preferential treatment in the allocation of resources for research, to remedy the injustices involved in the our practices concerning the inclusion of women in clinical studies.

Doubtless, critics of preferential treatment will respond to my conclusion here by complaining, as they often do, that it seems impossible for us to know for sure when we have done enough—that is, when programs of preferential treatment have been in place sufficiently long to complete their tasks of making amends for past and present injustices[37] and correcting for existing inequalities so they don't continue into the future.[38] These critics have a point; it will, indeed, be difficult to determine when programs of preferential treatment have achieved what they were designed to accomplish. However, we should not think that this difficulty undermines the acceptability of programs of preferential treatment. On the contrary, it is inappropriate for us to demand precise answers to questions about justice. As Aristotle says,

> Our discussion will be adequate if it achieves clarity within the limits of the subject matter. For precision cannot be expected in the treatment of all subjects alike. . . . Problems of what is noble and just, which politics examines, present so much variety and irregularity that . . . we must be satisfied to indicate the truth with a rough and general sketch.[39]

Furthermore, to object to the adoption of programs of prefer-ential treatment on the grounds that we won't know exactly when those programs have completed their mission is to send the wrong message to society, especially to members of the group that has suffered the injustices in question.[40] It is to say, "I know we cannot determine when we have doled out enough preferential treatment to correct for the injustices in question. So if we do anything, we risk doing too much. I'd rather refuse to remedy the injustices under discussion than risk depriving the dominant group in society of any more goods than is absolutely necessary." Justice simply cannot tolerate this kind of attitude. We must simply accept that precise answers cannot be given, and do the best we can to monitor the moral progress our remedies allow us to achieve.

Finally, we must address the question of who should be held responsible for making the changes necessary for securing justice for women. Of course, we cannot make these changes without the cooperation of everyone involved. For example, researchers must take the steps necessary to include women in their studies, to investigate whether the sex of the research subject is relevant to the condition or treatment being studied, and to avoid treating women's bodies as deviant or problematic compared to men's. Those who train researchers must instruct them about women's health needs, and should encourage more women to become researchers, since women researchers are likely to be more sensitive than men to women's health needs.

Ultimately, however, we must do more than call upon the cooperation of those involved in the pursuit of knowledge about women's health. The appropriate federal agencies must adopt regulations that implement the dictates of justice as I have outlined them in this paper. I cannot give an exhaustive summary of these dictates and their correlative regulations here, but they include the following: Our regulations must require researchers not only to include women in studies but to investigate whether the sex of the research subject is relevant to the condition or treatment being studied. They should encourage the study of women's health issues. They must require the presumption of the inclusion, not the exclusion, of women of childbearing age and pregnant women in studies. They must take the benefits research is likely to have for the health of women as a group (not just the individuals involved in the studies) into account in the risk-benefit assessments done to assess the merits of research proposals. They must insure that policies concerned with the protection of fetal health treat women and men consistently, and do not discriminate unjustly against women. And they must require the preferential treatment of women's health issues in the allocation of resources for research. I recognize that it will be politically difficult to secure the passage of such regulations. Nevertheless, justice demands that we do.[41]

NOTES

1. Throughout this paper I shall talk about women as a group. I realize that the group of women is not a homogeneous one; there are many subgroups, created by the multiple group memberships of individual women (e.g., memberships in a particular race, economic class, etc.). However, it is beyond the scope of this paper to do a fine-grained analysis of the ways in which our practices concerning the inclusion of women in clinical studies has affected women of particular subgroups. For some comments on these issues, see Susan Sherwin, "Women in Clinical Studies: A Feminist View," in this volume, a presentation to the March 24–25, 1993, workshop sponsored by the Institute of Medicine Committee on the Legal and Ethical Issues Relating to the Inclusion of Women in Clinical Studies (hereafter, simply the IOM workshop).

2. I shall use the terms "clinical research" and "clinical studies" interchangeably. The Institute of Medicine Committee on the Legal and Ethical Issues Relating to the Inclusion of Women in Clinical Studies defines the term "clinical studies" broadly to include, among other things, "epidemiological studies, health services research and outcomes research, as well as randomized clinical trials" (letter from Anna Mastroianni, Study Director, on file with author). Hence, I, too, shall use the term broadly.

3. See, for example, Rebecca Dresser, "Wanted: Single, White Male for Medical Research," *Hastings Center Report*, January–February 1992; Paul Cotton, "Examples Abound of Gaps in Medical Knowledge Because of Groups Excluded from Scientific Study," *Journal of the American Medical Association*, vol. 263, no. 8, Feb. 23, 1990; and Paul Cotton, "Is There Still Too Much Extrapolation From Data on Middle-aged White Men," *Journal of the American Medical Association*, vol. 263, no. 8, Feb. 23, 1990.

4. See Ruth Faden, Nancy Kass, and Deven McGraw, "Women as Vessels and Vectors: Lessons from the HIV Epidemic" (in press), for an excellent discussion of this problem.

5. See NIH/ADAMHA Inclusion of Minorities and Women as Subjects in Research: Grants and Cooperative Agreement Applications, 1992.

6. Cotton, "Is There Still Too Much Extrapolation From Data on Middle-aged White Men?" p. 1049; the quotation is from a letter to the General Accounting Office from Rep. Olympia Snowe and Rep. Patricia Schroeder (cochairs of the Congressional Caucus on Women's Issues), which Cotton quotes.

7. See *General Considerations for the Clinical Evaluation of Drugs*, U.S. Food and Drug Administration, 1977. On March 24, 1993, the FDA announced a change in policy concerning the inclusion of women of childbearing potential in drug trials. This change in policy is an attempt to switch the presumption from one of exclusion to one of inclusion.

8. E.L. Kinney et al., "Underrepresentation of Women in New Drug Trials," *Annals of Internal Medicine*, vol. 95, no. 4, 1981.

9. Dresser, p. 24.

10. Cotton, "Examples Abound of Gaps in Medical Knowledge Because of Groups Excluded From Scientific Study," pp. 1051, 1055.

11. See, for example, Faden et al.

12. Faden et al.

13. Ibid.

14. See Dresser, p. 27.

15. U.S. Public Health Service, "Report of the Public Health Service Task Force on Women's Health Issues", Public Health Reports, vol. 100, no. 1, 1985.

16. See, for example, Carol Weisman and Sandra Cassard "Health Consequences of Exclusion or Underrepresentation of Women in Clinical Studies," a presentation to the IOM workshop, in this volume; "What Doctors Don't Know About Women," Washington Post, Oct. 8, 1992; Gena Corea, The Invisible Epidemic: The Story of Women and AIDS (New York: Harper Collins Publishers, 1992); Faden et al.; and Margaret F. Jensvold et al., "Menstrual Cycle-Related Depressive Symptoms Treated with Variable Antidepressant Dosage," Journal of Women's Health volume 1, No. 2, 1992.

17. The phrase is from Iris Marion Young; see her Justice and the Politics of Difference (Princeton, N.J.: Princeton University Press, 1990).

18. Of course, the inclusion of women in studies could also have detrimental effects on the health of the women involved in the studies. However, I'm presuming here that (allowable) research has benefits, on balance, for the health of women (not just those included in the studies, but women as a group).

19. The general characterization of this aspect of oppression (which I provide in this sentence) owes much to Iris Young. See her Justice and the Politics of Difference, especially pp. 58–61. The fuller account of this aspect of oppression (in what follows here) is my own.

20. Michael S. Kimmel and Michael Messner, "Introduction," in Men's Lives, second edition, eds. Kimmel and Messner (New York: Macmillan, 1992), pp. 2–3.

21. Ibid., p. 2.

22. Some feminists reject this practice and use "she" as a gender-neutral pronoun. However, this is not standard usage. As far as I know, no one uses "woman" as a gender-neutral term meaning "person."

23. Note that individuals can belong to many different groups and so can suffer compound varieties of oppression (as do, e.g., black women), and so can be subordinate in more than one way. Or they can suffer some varieties of oppression while enjoying some varieties of privilege (as do, e.g., white women), and so can be dominant in one respect but subordinate in another.

24. But notice that they specify different aspects of our social conception of men and women than does false universalism. False universalism is a matter of conceiving of men in gender-neutral terms, as paradigmatic persons, and of women in terms of their gender, as problematic or inferior insofar as they are different from men. Gender norms specify what a "real" or "good" woman and man are like.

25. Iris Young denies that we can meaningfully speak of the distribution of abstract goods. See her Justice and the Politics of Difference, especially chapter 1. For further discussion of this point, see my review of this book in Ethics, vol. 103, No. 2, January 1993. Also, note that Young thinks we cannot give a purely distributive account of

dominance and subordination because she thinks we cannot meaningfully speak of the distribution of abstract goods like power. She agrees with the standard account that this aspect of oppression should be analyzed in terms of power imbalances. Thus my account here differs significantly from hers.

26. *Washington Post*, Oct. 8, 1992.

27. Researchers do not necessarily make conscious decisions to base their research on the conceptions of men and women given by our gender norms; individuals' participation in oppressive practices is often not a matter of conscious choice.

28. Gena Corea, *The Invisible Epidemic*, see especially the chapter entitled "July–November 1990." See also Faden et al.

29. See The National Commission for the Protection of Human Subjects of Biomedical and Behavioral Research, *Research on the Fetus: Report and Recommendations*, DHEW Publication No. (OS) 76-127, 1975; these recommendations were adopted as federal regulations in that year and still apply as such. I owe my familiarity with these regulations to the presentations given by Bonnie Steinbock and John Robertson at the IOM workshop, both entitled "Ethical Issues Related to the Inclusion of Pregnant Women in Clinical Trials," both in this volume. The regulations apply to studies involving actually pregnant women. However, at least until recently, similar regulations applied to women of childbearing potential who are not pregnant; see Vanessa Merton, "The Impact of Current Relevant Federal Regulations on the Inclusion of Female Subjects in Clinical Studies," a presentation for the above mentioned workshop, in this volume. On March 24, 1993, the FDA announced a change in policy concerning the inclusion of women of childbearing potential in drug trials. As I understand it, the policy change was motivated, at least in part, by a concern for the health of women as a group. See "FDA Ends Ban on Women in Drug Testing," 29.2231 *New York Times*, March 25, 1993.

30. We now face the possibility of weighing three different factors in our risk-benefit analyses to determine whether particular proposed studies would pose what we would deem to be acceptable risks to the individuals involved: (1) benefits (and risks) to the individual woman actually involved in the study; (2) benefits (and risks) to the individual fetuses actually involved in the study; and (3) benefits (and risks) the research could generate for the group of women as a whole (not only those actually involved in the study). Current policy has us take (1) and (2) into account. I here insist that we should take all three factors into account. Of course, doing so should modify the risk-benefit analysis from the way it is done now, so that benefits, not just to individual women in the study but to women generally, could justify taking some more (how much is an open moral question) risks with the health of the fetus involved than current policy justifies. On this point I strongly disagree with the positions endorsed by Steinbock and Robertson in their presentations to the IOM workshop (in this volume).

31. Until recently, FDA guidelines stated that women of childbearing potential should be excluded from drug trials in virtually all cases. The guidelines defined the class of women of childbearing potential as including women using contraception, sexually inactive women, women whose husbands are using contraception or have had vasectomies—essentially, all premenopausal women. See FDA, *General Considerations for the Clinical Evaluation of Drugs* (Washington, D.C.: U.S. Government Printing Office, FDA Publication 77-3040, 1977). The FDA recently announced a change in its guidelines on this issue; see "FDA Ends Ban on Women in Drug Testing," *New York*

Times, March 25, 1993.

32. I thank Vanessa Merton for reminding me of this point. See her "Impact of Current Relevant Regulations on the Inclusion of Female Subjects in Clinical Studies," a presentation to the IOM workshop, in this volume. See also Johnson and Fee, in this volume.

33. I borrow the phrase "cross-temporal perspective" from Thomas E. Hill Jr. See his "Message of Affirmative Action," reprinted in his *Autonomy and Self-Respect* (New York: Cambridge University Press, 1991).

34. Perhaps gender would be relevant to justice even apart from the context of an oppressive society. However, I cannot explore this possibility in this paper. For an interesting discussion of this issue, see Young's *Justice and the Politics of Difference;* Young develops a view of justice in which gender (and race, etc.) is relevant even apart from the context of oppression.

35. Men can be oppressed, but, in our society, they are not oppressed by virtue of being men. Instead, they are oppressed by virtue of their membership in other (oppressed) groups. So black men can be oppressed in virtue of being black, gay men can be oppressed in virtue of being gay, and so on.

36. Moreover, we should be wary about embracing any purportedly gender-neutral policies. As we have seen, important aspects of the oppression of women involve our social conception of them. As we have also seen, this social conception of women can influence what research gets done and what does not. In a society in which women tend to disappear from the conceptual scene when we think in gender-neutral terms, and in which, even when they are noticed, women's interests are taken to be less important than the interests of others because of their subordinate status, it will be difficult, at best, to insure that a purportedly gender-neutral policy of nondiscrimination is *truly* gender-neutral. And, as I have just shown, even truly gender-neutral policies are unacceptable from the point of view of justice.

37. Discussions of this objection to preferential treatment typically do not make this point in quite these terms. Instead, as I mentioned above, discussions of this "backward-looking" function of preferential treatment tend to characterize it as compensation to individuals for past injustices. As I also discussed above, I think it is more appropriate to frame the issue in terms of making amends to groups for past and present injustices.

38. For a presentation of this sort of objection to programs of preferential treatment, see Lisa Newton, "Reverse Discrimination as Unjustified," *Ethics*, vol. 83, 1973, pp. 308–312.

39. Aristotle, *Nichomachean Ethics*, translated by Martin Ostwald (Indianapolis: Bobbs-Merrill, 1962), I. 3, 1094b12–20.

40. I owe this insight to Thomas Hill; see his "Message of Affirmative Action."

41. I owe special thanks to Alisa Carse for valuable discussions about the issues contained in this paper; to Anna Mastroianni and Thelma Cox for their patient and cheerful assistance with my many questions and requests as I worked on this project; and to the participants at the March 24–25, 1993, workshop sponsored by the Institute of Medicine Committee on the Legal and Ethical Issues Relating to the Inclusion of Women in Clinical Studies, for stimulating discussion of a short presentation based on this paper, and of the issues involved in the exclusion of women from studies in general.

Women's Representation as Subjects in Clinical Studies: A Pilot Study of Research Published in *JAMA* in 1990 and 1992

Chloe E. Bird

In June 1990, the General Accounting Office reported that women have been and continue to be underrepresented in biomedical research populations (U.S. General Accounting Office 1990). However, researchers and policymakers continue to debate whether women are underrepresented as subjects in medical research. Both the debate and research on the question have tended to focus on clinical trials (Kinney et al., 1981; Halbreich and Carson, 1989; U.S. General Accounting Office, 1990; Dresser, 1992; Gurwitz, Col, and Avorn, 1992; Minkoff, Moreno, and Powderly, 1992; Bennett, 1993), but the issues of women's representation relate to clinical research as more broadly conceived. One consequence of the debate was the establishment of the Office of Research on Women's Health (ORWH) at the National Institutes of Health in September 1990 "to develop special initiatives to acquire vitally needed research data on women by increasing the participation both of women as subjects in clinical trials research and of institutions and investigators in performing research related to the health of women" (ORWH, 1991:67). Nevertheless, since the majority of medical studies which have an important bearing on clinical practice are not based on clinical trials, a thorough examination of women's representation in medical research needs to include the range of medical studies.

One reason that much of the debate over women's representation in medical research has focused on clinical trials is that past policies excluded women of childbearing age regardless of their pregnancy status or preference to avoid pregnancy, either through lifestyle or birth control. Recent changes in the federal Food and Drug Administration's (FDA) position regarding drug trials are intended to increase women's representation in those studies from which women were excluded in the past (Merkatz et al., 1993). The FDA has altered its policy that excluded most women with "childbearing potential" from the earliest phases of clinical trials. In addition, the FDA will provide formal guidance to drug developers emphasizing the need for women to be appropriately represented in clinical studies. However, the FDA's oversight responsibilities are restricted primarily to new drugs and medical devices; hence increased participation of women may be limited to these areas.

In order to evaluate whether women have been excluded from or underrepresented in clinical studies in general, we examined articles published in *The Journal of the American Medical Association (JAMA)* for 1990 and 1992. We selected *JAMA* because it is well respected and as a general medical journal, it presents a broad spectrum of clinical questions and reaches a wide audience. This report represents the preliminary results of a larger study designed to examine several major medical journals and to span publications over the past 15 years. While the results presented here are more narrowly construed, they represent the current state of the literature from a major general medical journal in the United States.

The analyses in this paper address the basic question: to what extent do recently published clinical studies include women as subjects? To address this question, we first classify the clinical studies by the percentage of female subjects included, the type of disease, gender(s) affected, basic design methodology, and the presence or absence of subgroup analysis based on gender and/or minority status. These classifications then permit us to examine:

• Is there any evidence that women are underrepresented compared to men in clinical studies of diseases that affect both genders?
• For studies based exclusively on one gender, to what extent does disease type necessitate the exclusive focus, either because the disease is gender-specific or because of its prevalence among the population?
• Among clinical studies that represent both genders and majority/minority subgroups, what evidence is there that subgroup analyses were performed?

While some researchers and policymakers have argued that representation of women in clinical studies is important for its own sake, most are concerned that the consequences of underrepresentation lead women to have poorer care (ORWH, 1991). There are several mechanisms by which this could occur. First, assuming that there are differences in the efficacy of the treatment for women and men, a gender bias in research can lead to a disproportionately lower or slower identification of effective treatment for women. For example, if women are not included in research, it may be wrongly assumed that the treatment is efficacious for them as well. Or, if a drug is not efficacious for men, a lack of research on women may deprive them of a possibly efficacious treatment.

Second, the lack of systematic collection of information about side effects among women owing to exclusion of women from early phases of clinical trials or from observational studies can lead to a slower recognition of their presence and form in women. To an important extent, side effects identified through the first stage of clinical studies, particularly clinical trials, appear more "legitimate" in subsequent appearances at a later stage presumably because they are more common and more important physiologically. Consequently, when side effects appear more commonly among women but are identified only in later stages of research, their appearance among women may help promote later attribution of problems in women to their being complainers or to psychological problems rather than to "real" effects. Third, whether or not there are actual gender-specific differences in efficacy, the exclusion of women from clinical studies may lead to uncertainty whether a treatment or problem applies to women and to reluctance among clinicians to apply a new therapy or diagnosis to women, resulting in a difference in access to care. Thus, findings of no significant gender differences are also important to women's medical care. Published medical studies provide the most credible scientific basis by which clinicians learn to treat their patients. Clinicians who perceive a lack of research on women for a particular disease or treatment can only extrapolate from studies of men and assume, perhaps wrongly, that a treatment may be equally applied.

METHODS

Sample

We examined all articles published in the "Original Contributions" section of *JAMA* during 1990 and 1992. By focusing on articles published in this section, we sought to avoid invited articles and opinion pieces. We included studies that examined a particular population (e.g., health care workers or Vietnam veterans) as well as both single-gender and non-gender-specific studies. Meta-analyses were excluded as well as articles that did not examine a health problem (e.g., articles examining gun ownership, the status of women physicians, or the total cost of universal precautions in a teaching hospital). We also excluded studies that lacked individual-level data (e.g., articles that compared hospital-, county-, or country-level data without demographic information on patients or respondents). (See the Appendix for a list of bases for exclusion.)

Data Collection

Owing to time constraints, the analyses are primarily based on the work of a single coder. A second coding of the data was completed for 92 of the articles (25.3 percent) in order to check the reliability of coding. Intercoder reliability based on three key variable—study design, women's representation, and presence of subgroup analysis by gender—was .98, .95, and .85, respectively. Inconsistencies were reexamined to determine the correct coding. In addition, half of the singly coded articles were rechecked by the same coder in order to ensure accurate coding.

Measures and Rules for Coding

In order to evaluate women's representation, we collected information on the proportion of respondents who were female and the extent of data analysis by gender. In addition, articles were classified in terms of study design, number of patients or respondents, disease or problem studied, average age of the respondents, and the extent of data analysis by race or ethnicity.[1] (Hereafter, we shall refer to the individuals from each study as respondents whether or not the study examined a patient population.)

We categorized the *percentage of respondents who were female* as follows: 0; 1 to 33 percent; 34 to 66 percent; 67 to 99 percent; and 100 percent. We categorized whether the data were *analyzed by gender* as follows: (1) no statistical analysis by gender reported; (2) no significant association between gender and the outcomes or dependent variables studied and no further statistical analysis by gender reported; (3) gender significantly associated with an outcome, no further analysis by gender reported; (4) controlled for gender in multivariate analyses, no further statistical analysis by gender reported; (5) controlled for gender in multivariate analyses and reported testing for gender interactions; (6) data analyzed separately by gender. These categories correspond roughly to the stringency with which the articles incorporate gender information.[2] (Hereafter, the term "outcome" refers broadly to the dependent variables in the studies examined.)

Study design was coded as follows: randomized controlled trial (including both placebo controlled trials and crossover studies), longitudinal, surveillance studies, cross-sectional studies, and case series. *Longitudinal studies* include both cohort and panel studies. *Surveillance studies* include those descriptive studies assessing the incidence and prevalence of a particular disease or condition over a particular timing period ranging from a brief outbreak to a decade or more. *Cross-sectional studies* include all studies where the data were collected at a single point in time except those examining the consequences of a common prior event, which were classified as longitudinal (e.g., a study of post traumatic stress among Vietnam War veterans). *Case series* refers to case studies of more than one respondent with a particular disease or disorder.

Seven articles included multiple sets of data reflecting different study types. For example, an article might include both a cross-sectional component and a case-controlled component. In order to provide a conservative estimate of whether women were underrepresented in clinical research and whether data for women were analyzed thoroughly, we coded each article that reported on multiple methods as using the highest level of any of the components for representing women. For example, if any component analyzed the data by gender, the entire article was coded as "6" and the other characteristics of the article were coded on the basis of that component.

Number of respondents refers to the number of individuals included in the primary analysis of an article. For example, in a case-controlled study, number of respondents includes the total number of people in the control and intervention groups. For a survey, number of respondents refers to the actual number of cases available for analysis rather than the original sample size; similarly for a longitudinal study, it refers to the number of respondents available in the final wave of data (those available at follow-up).

Diseases were classified on the basis of *Harrison's Principles of Internal Medicine* (Wilson et al., 1991) and *Internal Medicine Diagnosis and Therapy* (Stein, 1991). Articles that examined infectious diseases were always categorized as such whether or not the disease also fit into another category, such as reproductive disorders. Articles that examined both clinical and nonclinical aspects of a single disease were classified on the basis of the disease grouping. For example, an article which examined the cost effectiveness of misoprotal for prophylaxis against non-steroidal anti-inflammatory drug (NSAID)-induced gastrointestinal bleeding was classified as a musculoskeletal study because NSAIDs are used to treat musculoskeletal diseases or disorders. Articles that did not fit primarily into one internal medicine category were classified as *health services research* if the article examined issues of access to care, quality of care, practice guidelines, resource use, effects of insurance type, small area variation in treatment, or outcomes for multiple types of diseases. For example, one article examined small area variation in coronary angiography, carotid endarterectomy, and upper gastrointestinal endoscopy. Articles were classified as *public health* if they examined risk behaviors as outcomes, exposure to environmental toxins, the effect of public health education interventions, or the general health of a particular population (e.g., health status of Native American youth, health of children adopted from Romania).

Studies that examined non-gender-specific diseases using a single-gender sample were categorized by the primary *basis for excluding one gender*: prevalence (for example, the disease occurs disproportionately in one gender or the particular vector or risk factor of interest was gender-specific), convenience (for example, the population was veterans or prisoners, data gathering was easier in one gender, or the study was a secondary analysis of data from a gender-specific study), or no discernible rationale. We used a generous definition of prevalence, according to which we included all studies of diseases that are either more prevalent in one gender or for which there are variations in the manifestation of the disease by gender. Only studies of diseases not known to vary by gender were classified as studying a single gender owing to convenience sampling. Hereafter we use the terms "non-gender-specific" and "gender neutral" to refer to diseases that are reasonably common in both men and women.

For 1990 articles, we gathered information on whether racial or ethnic minorities were included in the study. The extent of analysis by race was based on a coding scheme parallel to that for gender.

ANALYSIS

First, to determine whether women have been excluded from medical studies, we examine the distribution of single-gender studies by whether or not the disease studied is gender-specific and, if not, the apparent rationale for using a single-gender population. Second, to evaluate the broader issue of whether women have been underrepresented in medical studies, we examine women's representation in studies of non-gender-specific diseases using two definitions of "underrepresentation of gender": (1) one gender is excluded from the study, and (2) one gender composes less than one-third of the sample. The former refers to the exclusion of men or women from studies of non-gender-specific disease, while the latter describes underrepresentation more leniently. Using these two definitions, we examine women's representation by study design, type of disease, and age of respondents. Third, we examine the extent to which studies that included both men and women examined the data by gender. Finally, we examine the extent to which data are examined by race or ethnicity.

RESULTS

In 1990 and 1992, *JAMA* published a total of 363 articles under the heading of original contributions.[3] Of these, 63 were excluded because they did not examine a health outcome, the data were not patient-level, or the study was a meta-analysis. (See the Appendix for a detailed list of reasons for exclusion.) Of the remaining 300 articles, 57 either did not report the percentage of women in the study sample or directed the reader elsewhere to learn such basic information about the sample.[4] (Twenty of these 57 articles, or 35.0 percent, provided indirect evidence that both genders had been included, for example, by inference from the analyses reported.) The present study examines the remaining 243 articles.

Have women been excluded from medical studies? In order to determine whether a higher proportion of gender-neutral problems have been studied using only men, we examined the 82 studies that included all male or all female respondents. Table 1 presents the distribution of articles involving only one gender as subjects, by whether or not the disease was gender-specific. There are two interesting features to note. First, among studies focusing on single-gender diseases, there were twice as many studies focusing on women's diseases compared to men's. One reason for the greater number of studies on women's diseases is the inclusion of studies focusing on pregnancy and childbirth.[5] Second, about 1 out of every 4 male-only studies was gender-specific, while 2 out of every 3 female-only studies were gender-specific.

Table 1. Distribution of Articles Examining Only One Gender

	Men		Women	
	N	%	N	%
Gender-specific diseases[a]	12	26.1	24	66.7
Non-gender-specific diseases	34	73.9	12	33.3
Total	46	100.0	36	100.0

[a]One of the studies categorized as male gender specific examined anal intraepithelial neoplasia and anal papillomivirus among male homosexuals with group IV HIV. Three of the studies categorized as male gender specific examined occupational health consequences for Vietnam veterans (one examined post traumatic stress, and two examined health consequences of herbicide exposure). All studies of breast cancer and benign breast disease were coded as female gender specific.

Is women's underrepresentation in studies of gender-neutral diseases explained by gender differences in disease prevalence? Table 2 shows the distribution of the 46 single-gender studies of gender-neutral diseases by the gender of respondents and the primary basis for excluding one gender. Overall, the choice of single-gender populations could be rationalized by either the prevalence of the disease or sampling convenience in most instances (87 percent). The remaining 13 percent of studies had no apparent rationale, either offered by the authors or inferred on the basis of the disease or site of study. This percentage was similar for male-only and female-only studies (12 percent vs. 17 percent). However, female-only and male-only studies appeared to differ systematically by whether the basis of the choice was disease prevalence (75 percent of female-only studies vs. 41 percent of male-only studies) or convenience (8 percent of female-only studies vs. 47 percent of male-only studies). Partial explanations for this imbalance were that 53 percent of all studies for which convenience was the primary basis examined the almost exclusively male veteran population and another 24 percent of these studies consisted of secondary analyses of single-gender studies which tended to be all-male.

Table 2. Distribution of Single-Gender Studies of Non-Gender-Specific Diseases by Gender and Rationale

Rationale	Male		Female		Total	
	N	%	N	%	N	%
Prevalence	14	41.2	9	75.0	23	50.0
Convenience	16	47.1	1	8.3	17	37.0
Neither	4	11.7	2	16.7	6	13.0
Total	34	100.0	12	100.0	46	100.0

Have women been underrepresented in studies of non-gender-specific diseases? Table 3 shows the distribution of the 207 articles that examined non-gender-specific diseases by the percentage of women in the sample. Women were excluded from 16.4 percent of studies and men were excluded from 5.8 percent. Using a broader definition of underrepresentation as consisting of any sample with one-third or fewer respondents of one gender, 37.2 percent of studies where both genders are relevant had unequal representation of women compared to 14.0 percent with unequal representation of men. Based on either definition, women were underrepresented in over 2.7 times as many studies of non-gender-specific diseases as men.

Do studies of gender-specific and non-gender-specific diseases differ significantly in terms of the age of respondents, sample size, or study methodology (see Table 4)? Studies of gender-specific diseases were significantly more likely to focus on working-age adults; 57 percent of studies of non-gender-specific diseases focused on working-age adults compared to 86.1 percent of the studies of gender-specific diseases.[6] Studies of gender-specific and non-gender-specific diseases did not differ significantly in sample size or methodology.

Table 3. Distribution of Articles by the Percentage of Women in the Sample for Non-Gender-Specific Diseases[a]

% of Women in Sample	Frequency	% of Studies
No women	34	16.4
1–33%	43	20.8
34–66%	101	48.8
67–99%	17	8.2
No men	12	5.8
Total	207	100.0

[a]Fifty-two articles are not included in this table because they reported neither the number nor the percentage of women in the sample. Of these, 23 either controlled for gender or reported whether there was a significant gender difference in the outcome.

Is women's underrepresentation in studies of non-gender-specific diseases limited to particular types of studies? Table 5 shows the distribution of articles by study design and proportion of women in the sample. There were three types of methodological designs, with at least 40 articles concerning gender-neutral diseases: cross-sectional (44), longitudinal (100), and random controlled trials (40). For all three types of designs, about 50 percent of the studies had samples with women representing between one-third and two-thirds of the subjects. Women were excluded from 6.8 percent of the cross-sectional studies, 18.0 percent of the longitudinal studies, and 25.0 percent of the random controlled trials. To compare the study methodologies, we calculated the ratio of the number of studies in which women were underrepresented compared to the number in which men were underrepresented. Among studies that excluded one gender, this ratio was .8 for cross-sectional studies, 3.6 for longitudinal studies, and 5.0 for random controlled trials. Using the lenient definition of underrepresentation, this ratio was 2.5 for cross-sectional studies, 2.8 for longitudinal studies, and 3.4 for random controlled trials. Using either definition, the women were most often underrepresented compared to men in randomized trials. The greatest differences in women's representation were between cross-sectional studies and randomized trials.

Table 4. Distribution of Articles by Age of Respondents, Sample Size, and Study Methodology (N = 243)

	Non-Gender-Specific Studies (N = 207)		Gender-Specific Studies (N = 36)	
	Frequency	%	Frequency	%
Age of Respondents				
Children (0–18)	17	8.5	1	2.8
Working-age adults (18–65)	118	57.0	31	86.1
Older adults (>65)	41	19.8	2	5.6
All ages	24	11.6	1	2.8
Not reported	7	3.4	1	2.8
Sample Size				
30 or less	10	4.8	3	8.3
31–100	23	11.1	7	19.4
101–300	39	18.8	5	13.9
301–1,000	48	23.2	8	22.2
1,001–10,000	52	25.1	7	19.4
10,001 or more	31	15.0	6	16.7
Not reported	4	1.9	0	0.0
Method				
Case series	6	2.9	0	0.0
Cross-sectional	44	21.3	8	22.2
Surveillance	17	8.2	2	5.6
Longitudinal	100	48.3	23	63.9
Random controlled trial	40	19.3	3	8.3

Table 5. Non-Gender-Specific Studies by Methodology and Women's Representation (N = 207)

	Percentage of women in the sample					
Method	0	1–33	34–66	67–99	100	Total
Case series	1	2	1	2	0	6
	16.7	33.3	16.7	33.3	0	2.9
	2.9	4.7	1.0	11.8	0	
Cross-sectional	3	11	24	1	5	44
	6.8	25.0	54.5	2.3	11.4	21.3
	8.8	25.6	23.8	5.9	41.7	
Surveillance	2	5	7	3	0	17
	11.8	29.4	41.2	17.6	0	8.2
	5.9	11.6	6.9	17.6	0	
Longitudinal	18	18	51	8	5	100
	18.0	18.0	51.0	8.0	5.0	48.1
	52.9	41.9	50.5	47.1	41.7	
Random con-	10	7	18	3	2	40
trolled trial	25.0	17.5	45.0	7.5	5.0	19.3
	29.4	16.3	17.8	17.6	16.7	
Total	34	43	101	17	12	207
	16.4	20.8	48.8	8.2	5.8	100.0

Are women less likely to be included in studies of particular types of diseases? Table 6 shows the distribution of articles on non-gender-specific diseases by disease type and women's representation. Because only a few disease categories have sufficient articles from which to generalize, we focus on the general patterns for disease types with 10 or more articles. The largest discrepancy occurred in studies of cardiovascular disease. Of the 38 articles on cardiovascular disease, women were excluded from 11 articles (28.9 percent of the articles), while men were excluded from none of the articles. In addition, women made up less than one-third of the cases in 24 articles (63.2 percent), while there were no articles in which men made up less than one-third of the cases. Similarly, of the 19 articles on dependency disorders and substance abuse, women were excluded from 4 articles (21 percent), while men were excluded from 1 article (5.3 percent). Using the second definition, women were underrepresented in 57.9 percent of the studies compared to 10.5 percent for men (a ratio of 5.5). Although women were slightly more likely than men to be studied exclusively in studies of infectious diseases (a ratio of .8), they were 1.7 times more likely to make up one-third or less of the sample.[7] In addition, women were somewhat likely to be underrepresented in articles on health services research, public health, and pulmonary diseases. Thus, women were substantially underrepresented across all disease types with 10 or more articles.

Table 6. Distribution of Articles on Non-Gender-Specific Diseases by Disease Type and Women's Representation

Disease Type	Percentage of Women in the Sample					
	0	1–33	34–66	67–99	100	Total
Cardiovascular	11	13	14	0	0	38
Dependency/substance abuse[a]	4	7	6	1	1	19
Endocrinology	1	0	2	1	1	5
Health services research	2	1	13	1	0	17
Hypertension	2	1	5	0	0	8
Infectious diseases	5	12	19	4	6	46
Metabolic disorders	4	0	6	0	2	12
Musculoskeletal disorders	0	0	3	5	1	9
Neurology	0	1	6	2	0	9
Oncology	0	1	2	0	0	3
Ophthalmology	1	0	1	0	1	3
Psychiatry	0	1	2	1	0	4
Public health	1	3	6	0	0	10
Pulmonary	1	2	6	1	0	10
Renal	1	1	5	0	0	7
Miscellaneous[b]	1	0	5	1	0	7
Total	34	43	101	17	12	207

[a]Dependency disorders and substance abuse includes articles on tobacco use.
[b]Miscellaneous includes two articles on neonatology and one article on each of the following: dermatology, gastroenterology, gerontology, hematology, and prenatal development.

Is women's underrepresentation limited to studies of a particular age group? Owing to the overlap in ages studied, we grouped articles into four categories:

those that examined children (0–18), those that primarily examined working age adults (19–65), those which primarily examined older adults (65 and up), and those studies that examined persons of all ages. Women were underrepresented in research in all categories (see Table 7). Much of the debate on women's representation has focused on the exclusion of women of childbearing age from clinical trials. Women were excluded from a larger proportion of studies of older adults than of working (or childbearing) age adults (19.5 percent compared to 16.1 percent). Among studies of working-age adults, women were excluded from 1.7 times as many studies and underrepresented in 2.1 times as many studies as men. By comparison, in studies of older adults, women were excluded from 8.0 times as many studies as men, and underrepresented in 3.0 times as many studies.

Table 7. Distribution of Studies of Non-Gender-Specific Diseases by Age Group of Respondents and Women's Representation (N = 208)

Age Group	Percentage of Women in the Sample					
	0	1–33%	34–66%	67–99%	100%	Total
Children (0–18)	1	3	13	0	0	17
Working-age adults (19–65)	19	26	52	10	11	118
Older adults (65 and up)	8	7	21	4	1	41
All ages	3	5	13	3	0	24

To what extent did studies that included both men and women examine the data by gender? Of the 161 articles that examined both men and women and reported the proportion of women in the sample, 48 (29.8 percent) reported no analysis by gender (see Table 8). These articles did not report bivariate associations between gender and the outcome variables and did not report controlling for gender in the analysis. An additional 29 articles (18.0 percent) indicated only whether gender was significantly associated with the outcomes studied. Of these, 16 reported that gender was not significantly associated with an outcome, and 13 reported that gender was significantly associated with an outcome. Forty articles (24.8 percent) controlled for gender in multivariate analyses, although not all of these reported their findings (e.g., gender was controlled for as a confounder and the results were not discussed). We cannot assume that gender was not significant in these analyses simply because results were not reported. Seven articles (4.3 percent) reported testing for some gender interactions, and 37 articles (23.0 percent) examined data for men and women separately. Thus, 27.3 percent of the articles reported testing whether the analyses found essentially the same results for men and women.[8] By contrast, 37.9 percent of the articles either reported no analysis by gender or reported significant bivariate associations of outcomes with gender and reported no further analysis.

Table 8. Frequencies for Level of Analysis by Gender for Studies That Examined Both Men and Women (N = 161)

Level of Analysis	Frequency	%
None	48	29.8
No significant association, and no further analysis	16	9.9
Significant association, and no further analysis	13	8.1
Controlled for gender in multivariate analysis, no further analysis	40	24.8
Tested for gender interactions	7	4.3
Analyzed data separately by gender	37	23.0
Total	161	99.9[a]

[a]Percentages do not total to 100.0 because of rounding.

Finally, to what extent did studies examine data by race or ethnicity? Although the analyses focus on gender, it is also important to consider whether minority women are excluded from or underrepresented in medical research. We examined analysis by race or ethnicity only for the 1990 data. Few studies included sufficient racial or ethnic minorities to analyze the data separately. Of the 148 articles examined, 106 (71.6 percent) had no analysis by race/ethnicity. Of the remaining studies, four examined minorities or ethnic groups (e.g., Hispanics) exclusively. The majority of studies that included a sizable proportion of minorities simply controlled for minority status as a confounder. In these cases, race was most often coded as a dummy variable (e.g., white/other, or black/other). However, some articles stated that the authors had controlled for race, but the measurement was not reported. Although the data on race and ethnicity may have been collapsed in order to obtain enough cases to test for significance, it is unlikely that racial differences are consistent such that all nonwhites or nonblacks are alike. Consequently, these studies provide only minimal information on racial or ethnic differences to clinicians treating minority patients.

Restricting the sample to studies of non-gender-specific diseases that reported women's representation, there were data on race/ethnicity for 95 studies. Among these studies, 67 (70.5 percent) reported no analysis by race. Eleven studies controlled for race/ethnicity in multivariate analyses. One study tested for race/ethnicity interactions and 7 studies analyzed the data separately by race. Thus only 8 (8.4 percent) reported substantial analysis by race and 19 (20.0 percent) reported analysis beyond bivariate associations. Of these 19 studies, 3 examined men exclusively and 2 examined women exclusively. Despite awareness in differences in the incidence and prevalence of certain diseases in minorities, and in some cases of differences in pharmacological actions of drugs, few studies reported even minimal analysis by race or ethnicity.

SUMMARY AND DISCUSSION

The results indicate that women are underrepresented in medical studies more often than men. Of studies excluding women, nearly three quarters examined diseases that are not gender-specific, compared to one-third of studies that excluded men. Among studies of non-gender-specific diseases, women were underrepresented in 2.7 times as many studies as men, whether underrepresentation is defined as exclusion or as representing one-third or less of the sample. Women's representation varied by study methodology: women were excluded from randomized clinical trials and longitudinal studies substantially more often than from cross-sectional studies (3.7 and 2.6 times, respectively). However, the problem of women's exclusion was not isolated to any one methodology. Of those disease types with sufficient articles for comparison, women were most often excluded from and underrepresented in studies of cardiovascular disease, dependency disorders/substance abuse, and studies of infectious disease. Finally, women's underrepresentation varied by age group. The greatest disparity in women's representation was in studies of older adults, where women were excluded 8.0 times as often as men and underrepresented 3.0 times as often as men. Women's underrepresentation in studies of working-age adults may be partially explained by fetal protection policies. However, since women outnumber men by 1.49 to 1.00 among people age 65 and over in the U.S. population, the high levels of women's underrepresentation compared to men in studies of older adults were not expected (U.S. Bureau of the Census, 1993).

Among studies that examined respondents of only one gender, two-thirds of the studies of women were of gender-specific diseases compared to one-quarter of the studies of men. Similarly, in single-gender studies of diseases that affect both men and women, most studies of women were due to gender differences in the prevalence of the disease. By comparison, nearly half of the male-only studies of non-gender-specific diseases simply examined a sample of convenience. These findings suggest that one important reason for a tendency for male-only studies to predominate is the differential opportunity for men to be in positions where clinical studies are likely to be funded and carried out (for example, receiving treatment in a Veterans Administration medical center or as a member of the armed services or as a prisoner), which in turn can create further imbalance as researchers seek to take advantage of databases already collected. Perhaps one way to redress this source of gender imbalance in clinical studies is to fund studies of populations where women predominate (e.g., nursing home residents, hospital employees, or primary grade teachers).

In addition to the underrepresentation of women in medical research on non-gender-specific diseases, data from studies that included both men and women were underanalyzed for gender differences. Even those studies that are reasonably well balanced by gender often completely neglect to examine, or perhaps only to report, effects of gender on the outcomes of interest. Among articles that examined both genders, 29.8 percent reported no analysis by gender. An additional 8.1 percent reported significant bivariate associations between gender and outcome variables but no further analysis by gender.

It is unclear from the articles why many studies that included both genders did not report any analysis by gender. The samples may have included either too few women or too few men to test for significant gender differences (one consequence of underrepresenting either gender in a study). Authors may have chosen not to report findings that were not significant, or editors and reviewers may have encouraged or required authors to eliminate the discussion of nonsignificant findings. In fact, authors of some studies that reported minimal analysis of the data by gender may have conducted but not reported more thorough examinations of the data by gender. However, we cannot assume that articles which do not report gender differences tested for such differences and found them to be nonsignificant.[9] Whether or not such analyses are missing because the researchers or the editors found them to be unimportant, the information fails to enter the scientific literature. For women and for clinicians, it would be valuable to know that researchers found a particular treatment to work as well in women as in men.

Determining that there is no significant bivariate relationship between gender and the outcomes of interest is not an adequate basis for removing gender from further analysis. Certain health problems as well as certain treatments affect women differently than men. The reasons for these differences may be biological, behavioral, social, or some combination of the three. Unless gender is controlled for in a multivariate analysis, underlying differences may be overlooked (Hardy, 1993).[10] For example, age differences between women and men in the sample may confound the effects of gender on the outcome. Without testing the effect of gender in a multivariate analysis, it is impossible to ascertain whether gender differences or the lack thereof are due to other intervening or confounding factors. Even when researchers controlled for gender in multivariate analyses as a confounder, many did not report the effect of gender or report testing for interactions. In addition, many randomized clinical trials and case-controlled studies avoided examining the effect of gender, stratifying their samples to obtain equal representation of women in the control and intervention groups. For example, in a controlled trial of buprenorphine treatment for opioid dependence, Johnson, Jaffe, and Fudala (1992:2752) specifically state: "Gender differences have been reported to influence retention in methadone maintenance and therapeutic community treatment programs. Also since the present study incorporated fixed dosage regimens, potential pharmacokinetic differences due to gender were controlled by stratification [references omitted]." The authors make no further references to gender in the remainder of the article. Although the practice of controlling for gender differences by stratification is effective in assessing the general efficacy of a treatment regime, it is still valuable to assess gender differences and the findings, particularly since stratification is used when gender differences are expected. A number of other studies used the same technique, but at least Johnson and his colleagues acknowledged their rationale. Clearly, the practice of stratifying the sample by gender with no further analysis can undermine the benefits to women of being included in medical research.

Owing to the underanalysis or reporting of findings on women's health and of possible gender differences in health, an important contribution to understanding women's health and medical treatment comes from studies which are predominantly or exclusively of women, such as the Nurses' Health Study (Colditz, 1990; Hankinson et al., 1992; Romieu et al., 1989). In a pair of articles reported in *JAMA* issues analyzed for the present article, researchers from the nurses' and physicians' health studies published parallel research on the effects of cigarette smoking on the risk of cataracts for women and men. The simultaneous publication of these two articles offers a valuable example of overcoming the limitations of single-gender studies while gaining all the benefits of such studies.[11] Single-gender studies such as these allow researchers to focus on gender-specific problems and side effects. For example, the side effects of antihypertensive therapy for men included problems in obtaining and maintaining an erection and problems in ejaculation (Croog et al., 1986). Studies of men which determine how to avoid these side effects may not be appropriately generalized to women, as a treatment which causes sexual dysfunction in men may have fewer or less distressing side effects in women. Thus the best solution to women's underrepresentation in medical studies is not necessarily to mandate balanced representation in every study. Because of the unique benefits of single-gender studies, a preferable solution is to obtain a balance whereby single-gender studies are conducted as often among women as among men.

The present study examined only articles published in two recent years of *JAMA*. The findings suggest a need to examine the medical literature more broadly over time and across journals. In particular, the small sample size provided only limited indications of whether women are underrepresented in studies of particular diseases. Several additional questions should be addressed in a broader examination of the medical literature. Does women's representation vary by whether studies are patient or population based or whether respondents were selected to be representative or a sample of convenience? Research methods could be examined with greater detail than in the present study. For example, women's representation may vary by whether studies are interventions or observational. Finally, to what extent are women and men equally represented in studies that address the leading life-threatening and disabling diseases? Clearly one goal is to have a balance of studies dealing with the important health problems of both women and men.

Recently, medical researchers have moved from a narrow interest in biological explanations of differences in men's and women's health to a broader examination of how gender differences in health may be acquired through differences in the behaviors or treatment of men and women throughout their lives. Recognizing that differences may have social as well as biological origins increases the need for analysis of data by gender. In order to separate out the effects of social and biological factors, it is necessary to analyze the data by gender and to control for social variables as well. By failing to thoroughly examine gender differences, even in those studies which included both men and women, researchers fail to address either biological or acquired differences.

A more subtle implication of the underrepresentation of women in medical research which is rarely discussed is that men could also benefit from more inclusive medical research. Because medical research is advanced by studying what it is to be human and how the human body responds to both diseases and treatments, to overemphasize men as subjects may disadvantage men as well as women. Men may benefit from research on women which identifies advantages and disadvantages of women's biology. For example, one study in the sample examined the effects of female sex hormones on cancer survival for both men and women. In other words, a thorough understanding of men's and women's physiological responses to treatment may lead to better medical treatments for both men and women.

Women cannot necessarily take advantage of health recommendations that have emerged from men-only research studies (Dresser, 1992). Medical research provides the information necessary to tailor medical treatments to individual patients, particularly in the case of drug therapy (Kinney et al., 1981). Whether women are excluded from research in order to protect potential developing fetuses or simply because of the use of convenience samples (as in the eight studies in the sample which were conducted at Veterans Administration hospitals, none of which examined a gender-specific health problem), women lose opportunities to participate in clinical research. As individuals, the loss of opportunity may or may not be important. However, if data gathered primarily or exclusively from studies of men cannot be reliably generalized to women, then women as a group lose access to efficacious medical care. Similarly, clinicians do not gain the information necessary to provide their female patients with informed medical advice. Healy (1991) referred to the consequences of this lack of information about women's treatment as the Yentl syndrome, which she claims has resulted in less aggressive early treatment of women with cardiovascular disease. Findings of significant differences in women's and men's responses to particular treatments, incidence of side effects and the like, as well as findings of no significant gender differences, all contribute to clinicians' ability to treat their patients. Thus, the findings that women are underrepresented in medical studies and that in studies which include women, analysis by gender is either not done or not reported, have a significant impact on women's health care.

***

I would like to thank Matthew M. Wise for assistance in collecting and coding the data, and Allen M. Fremont and Harold Swartz for assistance in classifying the diseases. I also thank Ben Amick, Elizabeth Goodman, Kathy Lasch, Debra Lerner, Sol Levine, Ed Schor, Diana Chapman Walsh, and especially Ann Barry Flood for commenting on earlier drafts of this manuscript.

***

APPENDIX: REASONS FOR EXCLUDING ARTICLES FROM THE ANALYSES

Unit of Analysis

Methadone treatment programs
Hospital service area
County-level data only
Foods in the refrigerators of listeriosis patients
Lyme disease serology
Authors
Health/body building magazines
Episode data with no demographic information on patients
Facility

Comparison of lab diagnostic techniques with no demographic data
Prescription orders for hospitalized patients
Lung cells

Topic

Factors influencing publication
House officers' responses to hypothetical cases
Reducing the number of uninsured by subsidizing employer-based insurance
Factors that prompt families to file malpractice claims
Pediatricians' reasons for not participating in Medicaid
Comparison of assessments of quality of care
Evaluation of malpractice insurance costs
Survey of gun ownership
Primary care physicians' responses to domestic violence
Primary care physicians' attitudes toward corporeal punishment
Residents' attitudes toward or of persons with AIDS
Treatment of medical students
Medical reimbursement accuracy
Physician retention by the NHS Corps compared to other rural physicians
Which medical schools produce rural physicians
Hospital leaders' opinions of HCFA mortality data
Effects of medical student indebtedness and repayment on residents' cash flow
Understanding recent growth in Medicare physician expenditures
Physician reporting of adverse drug effects
Prevalence of reading disability in children
Attitudes of internal medicine faculty toward drug representatives
Status of women in an academic medical center
HIV testing policies at hospitals

Method of Analysis

Computer model of CHD primary prevention
Decision analysis study using hypothetical cohorts of women with breast cancer
Meta-analysis of randomized controlled trials for myocardial infarction
Literature review on the exclusion of older women from controlled trials
regarding acute myocardial infarction
Reanalysis of three previous studies
Meta-analysis on depression
Review of four previous studies
Computer simulation based on meta-analysis
Projection of trends based on review of the literature

Analysis of hypothetical data
Meta-analysis
Literature review on the cost effectiveness of treating high cholesterol with drugs

Some studies could have been excluded for multiple reasons. Some studies are not included in this list because they duplicate an exact reason given.

REFERENCES

Aiken, Leona S. and Stephen G. West. *Multiple Regression: Testing and Interpreting Interactions.* Newbury Park, CA: Sage (1991).

Bennett, J. Claude. "Inclusion of Women in Clinical Trials Policies for Population Subgroups." *New England Journal of Medicine* 329(4):288–292 (1993).

Colditz, G. A. "The Nurses' Health Study: Findings during 10 Years of Follow-up of a Cohort of U.S. Women." *Current Problems in Obstetrics, Gynecology, and Fertility* 13:129–174 (1990).

Croog, Sydney H., Sol Levine, Marcia A. Testa, Byron Brown, Christopher J. Bulpitt, C. David Jenkins, Gerald L. Klerman, and Gordon H. Williams. "The Effects of Antihypertensive Therapy on the Quality of Life." *New England Journal of Medicine* 314:1657–1664 (1986).

Dresser, Rebecca. "Wanted: Single, White Male for Medical Research." *Hastings Center Report* 221:24–29 (1992).

Gurwitz, Jerry H., Nananda F. Col, and Jerry Avorn. "The Exclusion of the Elderly and Women from Clinical Trials in Acute Myocardial Infarction." *Journal of the American Medical Association* 268(11):1417–1422 (1992).

Halbreich, Uriel and Stanley W Carson. "Drug Studies in Women of Childbearing Age: Ethical and Methodological Considerations." *Journal of Clinical Psychopharmacology* 9(5):328333 (1989).

Hankinson, S. E., W. C. Willett, G. A. Colditz, J. Seddon, B. Rosner, F. E. Speizer, and M. J. Stampfer. "A Prospective Study of Nutrient Intake and Risk of Cataract Extraction in Women." *British Medical Journal* 93:13–18 (1992).

Hardy, Melissa A. *Regression with Dummy Variables.* Sage University Paper Series on Quantitative Applications in the Social Sciences. Series no. 07-093. Newbury Park, CA: Sage (1993).

Healy, Bernadine. "The Yentl Syndrome." *The New England Journal of Medicine* 325(4):274–276 (1991).

Johnson, Rolley E., Jerome H. Jaffe, and Paul J. Fudala. "A Controlled Trial of Buprenorphine Treatment for Opioid Dependence." *Journal of the American Medical Association* 267(20):2750–2755 (1992).

Kinney, Evlin L., Joanne Trautmann, Jay Alexander Gold, Elliot S. Vesell, and Robert Zelis. "Underrepresentation of Women in New Drug Trials." *Annals of Internal Medicine* 95(4):495–499 (1981).

Merkatz, Ruth B., Robert Temple, Solomon Sobel, Karyn Feiden, David A. Kessler, and the Working Group on Women in Clinical Trials. "Women in Clinical Trials of New Drugs: A Change in Food and Drug Administration Policy." *New England Journal of Medicine* 329(4):292–296 (1993).

Minkoff, Howard, Jonathan D. Moreno, and Kathleen R. Powderly. 1992. "Fetal Protection and Women's Access to Clinical Trials." *Journal of Women's Health* 1(2):137–140.

Office of Research on Women's Health (ORWH). *Report of the National Institutes of Health: Opportunities for Research on Women's Health.* Washington, DC: National Institutes of Health (1991).

Romieu, I., W. C. Willett, G. A. Colditz, M. J. Stampfer, B. Rosner, C. H. Hennekens, and F. E. Speizer. "A Prospective Study of Oral Contraceptive Use and the Risk of Breast Cancer in Women." *Journal of the National Cancer Institute* 81:1313–1321 (1989).

Stein, Jay H. *Internal Medicine Diagnoses and Therapy.* Lange Clinical Manual. Appleton and Lange: Norwalk (1991).

U.S. Bureau of the Census. *1990 Census of Population and Housing, Summary Tape File 3.* Washington, DC: U. S. Government Printing Office (1993).

U.S. General Accounting Office. Statement of Mark Nadel, National Institutes of Health: *Problems in Implementing Policy on Women in Study Populations.* Bethesda, MD: National Institutes of Health (June 18, 1990).

Wilson, Jean D., Eugene Braunwald, Kurt J. Isselbacher, Robert G. Petersdorf, Joseph B. Martin, Anthony S. Fauci, Richard K. Root. *Harrison's Principles of Internal Medicine.* New York: McGraw-Hill (1991).

NOTES

1. We attempted to code whether the data were collected at a single or multiple centers. Such information is most relevant for patient studies or studies with medical tests or interventions rather than community-based studies. On further examination we found two separate issues in the case of surveys. Surveys and surveillance data are often based on one or more communities or states, or a national sample. However, some studies, such as the Physicians' and Nurses' Health Studies, are a combination of surveys, medical examinations, and interventions. Further refinement of our coding scheme is necessary to examine whether these issues are associated with women's representation in medical studies.

2. Testing for all possible interactions between the effect of gender and other variables in the analysis is equivalent to analyzing the data separately (Aiken and West 1991). However, we found no instances where the authors clearly indicated that all possible gender interactions were tested. More often, authors reported testing for an interaction between gender and one or more key variables.

3. Of the 96 issues published in 1990 and 1992, nine issues did not include any original contributions, and one issue was devoted to MOS (Medical Outcomes Study) research. The latter included eight related articles, all in the original contributions section. Of these eight articles, one introduced and one concluded the series and two dealt solely with the methodology of the overall study. The remaining four articles all

focused on health service research and used gender and at times an age/gender interaction as one of a number of controls for case mix. These four articles referred to the introductory pieces for information on the sample. Unlike other articles that refer to information elsewhere, the reader can reasonably be assumed to have the entire issue available and therefore to have immediate access to the information. Because this is a unique situation among the journal issues studied, we have excluded these articles from the analysis. Although these four articles represent over one percent of the sample, our findings are strong enough that the addition of these articles will not significantly affect the results.

4. Wherever sufficient data were provided in the article to calculate the percentage of women in the study sample, we did so.

5. Three of the 24 female gender-specific studies examined pregnancy and an additional four examined reproductive health, compared with one male gender-specific study of reproductive health.

6. We chose the term "working age" to refer to adults ages 19 to 65 rather than the term "child-bearing age" which is typically used to refer to women between the ages of menarche and menopause. An accurate range for defining child-bearing age would have a lower beginning and end.

7. All of the non-gender-specific infectious disease studies that focused exclusively on one gender examined sexually transmitted diseases.

8. It is necessary to keep in mind that some of the studies did not conduct any multivariate analyses. Some surveillance studies simply reported the demographics, prevalence, and incidence of a particular disease or disorder and did not conduct further analysis.

9. Another possibility is that authors found significant gender differences which they intend to publish elsewhere in a separate article.

10. Whereas the zero-order correlation between gender and a particular health outcome contrasts the average outcome (or risk) for women and men, the first-order partial correlation coefficient controls for other factors expected to affect the outcome (or risk of the outcome).

11. Of the single-gender articles we examined, five were based on the Nurse's Health Study, three were based on the Physician's Health Study, and an additional eight were conducted at the VA.

Racial Differentials in Medical Care: Implications for Research on Women

Vanessa Northington Gamble and Bonnie Ellen Blustein

Federal guidelines now call for the inclusion of women in clinical studies unless a compelling reason is given for their exclusion. Initiatives to recruit women must not forget the diversity of women. Issues of race and ethnicity cannot be neglected. The purpose of this report is to examine the implications of racial differences on research involving women. It will focus primarily on African Americans. The report is divided into four sections. The first section explores definitions of race and the problems associated with using race as a variable in medical research. The second part analyzes how issues of race and racism have influenced past research efforts. It specifically concentrates on the fertility and osteoporosis literature. The third section studies an important obstacle to the inclusion of women of color in medical research—historically based distrust. The final part offers some recommendations about how racial differences in studies should be conceptualized.

The Construction of Race: An Historical Perspective

Over the last two decades, concepts of race have come under increasingly sophisticated analysis. Historians, sociologists, and philosophers have joined colleagues in the biomedical sciences and anthropology in the attempt to refine or critique these ideas. Interdisciplinary studies have made plain that "race" is often used casually and unreflectively in ways that may seem intuitively obvious but are profoundly flawed. Historian Evelyn Brooks Higginbotham aptly describes this view. She writes, "When we talk about the concept of race, most people believe that they know it when they see it but arrive at nothing short of confusion when pressed to define it."[1] But in the context of over 250 years of the mixing of gene pools in the United States, race is not always self-evident. As policies are developed and implemented to include more women of color in clinical trials, it is critical that the distinctions and implications of interpretations of race be more clearly scrutinized.

Concepts of race have evolved and changed since natural scientists first began in the seventeenth century to categorize human beings according to physical attributes. Indeed no consensus even exists among physical anthropologists, biologists, and social scientists about the definitions of race. There is, however, a legacy of debate, confusion, and controversy surrounding the meaning of the term. Divergent interpretations have centered primarily on whether race should be considered a biological construct or a sociological one. Biological constructionists hold that races are genetic entities that are fixed, immutable, and genetically determined. Different populations can be distinguished by distinctive traits that are inherited such as skin color, body build, facial features, and cephalic index. Skin color is the most common criterion used to classify race. Race is often viewed as synonymous with skin color. Thus, a phenotypic attribute is seen as an accurate measure of genotypic differences between human beings.

The social construction model holds that race is a social, historical, and political entity without any essential biological coherence. It is not a natural, fixed category; rather it has been created by society to recognize difference and establish social relationships. Race is viewed as a "highly contested representation of relations of power between social categories by which individuals are identified and identify themselves."[2] Therefore it cannot be understood outside of its historical and social context.

A historical examination of the concept of race clearly challenges the validity of the biological concept of race. Racial classification has been and continues to be an elusive concept. The accepted number of races, for example, has not been constant. It has varied between three and dozens and have included Jewish, Nordic, Amerindian, African, Alpine, and European races. The Swedish botanist Carol von Linneaus, in his classic work *Systematic Naturae* (1735) grouped humans into four "varieties"—white, red, yellow, and black. He based his taxonomy on skin color and physiognomy and then correlated these traits with temperament and personality type. In 1749, George Buffon, the naturalist who is credited with the use of the term "race" to describe human variation, maintained that there were six races. He used skin color, stature, and physique as the criteria for racial designation. Over 200 years later, in 1950, W.S. Boyd used blood group data to designate six races which he later revised into 13.[3]

Cross-cultural and historical studies have revealed changing, arbitrary, and inconsistent definitions of race.[4] These studies provide additional ammunition against the argument that races are biologically determined categories. Furthermore, they underscore the ways in which social, political, and cultural factors have influenced racial classification. Definitions of race differ according to geography. The same person defined as black in the United States may be considered "colored" in South Africa. Even in the United States, definitions of race have not been static. By the early twentieth century many states—in part as antimiscegenation measures—had adopted numerous criteria to legally assign race. One of the most common gauges was the "traceable amount rule" or "one drop rule," according to which a single drop of "black blood" made one black. The varying legal definitions of race in one state, Louisiana, illustrate the arbitrariness of racial classifications. The state followed the "one drop rule" until 1970 when it adopted more than one 1/32 black as the criterion for blackness. This law stood until 1983,when the legislature gave parents the right to designate the race of newborns.

Federal criteria to designate race also reveal vagueness and inconsistency. The situation of biracial children is illustrative of the continued ambiguities. The growing number of such children raises the question as to how they should be classified in federal health statistics. In 1989 the National Center for Health Statistics (NCHS) decided to tabulate new births by the race of the mother. Previously, in the tradition of the one-drop rule, it had used the race of the nonwhite parent as the determinant. It should be noted that scientific evidence did not guide either of the NCHS policies.

In a 1992 *JAMA* article, epidemiologist Robert A. Hahn analyzed the dilemmas associated with the collection of federal health statistics on racial and ethnic groups in the United States.[5] These difficulties raise profound question for medical research and clinical medicine. Hahn critiqued the assumptions underlying federal health statistics on racial and ethnic groups and questioned their validity. He stated that the accuracy of these statistics rested on logical assumptions that include the following: (1) The categories of "race"' and "ethnicity" are consistently defined and ascertained by federal data collection agencies. (2) Racial and ethnic categories are understood by the populations questioned. (3) Survey enumeration, participation, and response rates are high and similar for all racial and ethnic populations. (4) Individual responses to questions of racial and ethnic identity are consistent in different surveys and different times.

Hahn analyzed each of these assumptions and found that long standing conceptual difficulties in the definition of race and ethnicity challenged their validity. For example, he found that the terminology and definition of race differed from agency to agency. Agencies used separate sources and inconsistent procedures to categorize race including policy directives, self determination, and observer perception. Therefore, the biracial child classified as white by the NCHS might be classified as black by the Census Bureau, which uses self-identification as the basis for racial designation. In another example, Hahn illustrated that with different indicators, estimates of the 1970 Hispanic population ranged from 5.2 million (persons of Hispanic heritage) to 9.6 million (persons using the Spanish language).

The establishment of public health policy and the setting of medical research agendas are influenced by the morbidity and mortality rates of different racial and ethnic groups. Accurate statistical information is a key component in the development of these programs. As a step toward the improvement of federal health data, Hahn urged researchers to use more precision in their definitions of race and ethnicity.

In recent years there has been a growing trend to reject biological notions of race. For example, 40 years ago the United Nations Educational, Scientific and Cultural Organization (UNESCO) launched a major publicity campaign promoting the idea that "race is less a biological fact than a social myth." [6] Criticisms of the biological construction of race have increasingly grown since the initiation of this campaign. The voices of opposition have come from numerous disciplines, including biology, anthropology, and medicine. The views of the critics are aptly summarized by scientists Richard Lewontin, Stephen Rose, and Leon Kamin, who in 1984 wrote, "Any use of racial categories must take its justification from some other source than biology." [7] Physical anthropology, from its origins in the nineteenth century through the middle of the twentieth century, was based on the central assumption of the existence of the "'pure race' as an assemblage of traits manifest in every individual race member, essentially unchanged by time or circumstance." [8] But even within this profession, the current trend is to reject the proposition that distinct races exist within the human species and consequently to disavow biological concepts of race. Anthropologist Fatimah Jackson in a 1992 article about the use of race and ethnicity as biological constructs attributes this trend to a growing recognition by her colleagues of "the difficulty of making valid taxonomic assessments in long-lived, sexually reproducing, socially complex, and highly mobile species such as Homo sapiens." [9]

The traditional medical and public health view has been to interpret race as a biological and genetic category. This frequently takes the form of attributing observed differences in health status to inherent putatively "racial" characteristics. However, a growing number of researchers have begun to challenge this traditional perspective. They criticize the practice of interpreting racial differentials in health status as primarily the expression of biological factors. They contend that social factors must also be taken into consideration and that the focus on biological considerations obscures the importance of sociological and political ones. As cardiologist Richard Cooper has argued, "in the biologic sense there are no such things as races . . . the concept of race is itself a social category . . . [and] health status of racial groups should be viewed within this context." In particular, he explains, "black people in this society are imprisoned by institutional racism; this is the attribute of blackness which at bottom determines their health status."[10]   Cooper and other authors have criticized the tendency to conflate race with class and to use race as the dominant measure of health disparities.[11] This practice is compounded by the fact that the United States does not collect health statistics by class. Dr. Vicente Navarro, a prominent health policy analyst, asserts that health differentials cannot be explained solely by looking at race—class must also be taken into account. "The publication of health statistics in racial terms," he states, "assumes that white unskilled workers have more in common with white lawyers, for example, than with black unskilled workers."[12]

Criticism of the application of the biological model to medicine and public also focuses on the notion that race, that is, skin color, is an accurate measure of the biological differences between human beings. As Richard Cooper has pointed out:

> To classify on the basis of skin color arbitrarily assigns primary importance to that characteristic and forces all others to be ignored. Is there any reason to believe that variations in skin color subsume all, or any, biologically important human variation? The Masai, pygmies of the African rain forest, inhabitants of southern India, Australian aborigines, and natives of the Amazon are all dark-skinned: Are they members of the same race?[13]

Opponents also criticize the assumption in the biological model that associates the genes for skin color with those that affect health. Drs. Newton G. Osborne and Marvin D. Feit outlined this position in a 1992 *JAMA* article. They wrote:

> When race is used as a variable in research, there is a tendency to assume that the results obtained are a manifestation of the biology of racial differences; race as a variable implies that a genetic reason may explain differences in incidence, severity, or outcome of medical conditions. Researchers, without saying so, lead readers to assume that certain racial groups have a special predisposition, risk, or susceptibility to the illnesses studied. Since this presupposition is seldom warranted, this kind of comparison may be taken to represent a subtle form of racism.[14]

Of course biological factors cannot be dismissed when we analyze the health status of various racial and ethnic groups. Various genetic diseases are more prominent in particular racial and ethnic groups. Racial and ethnic differences in responses to drug therapies have also been ascertained. However, a close analysis of these cases demonstrates that biological considerations may not be as clear-cut as they initially appear. For example, medical historian Keith Wailoo has shown how sickle-cell anemia was defined as a "black" disease in the 1920s on the basis of half a dozen cases—all of which involved persons of obviously mixed African and European ancestry. The disease, however, is not limited exclusively to African Americans. It is also prevalent among people of Mediterranean, Middle Eastern, and East Indian ancestry.[15] In a move that once again underscores the problems of racial classification, a panel assembled by the Agency for Health Care Policy and Research recently urged that all newborns—not just black ones—be screened for sickle cell disease.[16] The chair of the panel, Dr. Jeanne A. Smith, pointed out that racially targeted screening would miss many with sickle cell disease. She noted, "Because of mixing of the gene pool, it's not always possible to be certain of an individual's racial or ethnic background by physical appearance, surname or self report." In other words, America's mixed gene widens the risk for the disease.

Recent pharmacological research has discovered differences between racial and ethnic groups in drug metabolism rates, clinical drug responses, and side effects.[17] Black patients with hypertension, it has been found, respond better to treatment with thiazides than with beta blockers. Preliminary studies have also indicated that smaller doses of haldol are needed to effectively treat Asian patients with schizophrenia. Much of this work has focused on the pharmacogenetics of drug metabolism. However, an emphasis on this area should not blind us to the effects of environmental and social factors, as the controversy surrounding a 1991 study of the effects of zidovudine (AZT) on HIV positive men clearly demonstrates. The study, conducted over a four year period, examined the effects of early therapy with the drug on 338 men—220 whites and 118 African Americans and Latinos. Its findings suggested that no benefit would be gained from early AZT therapy in African Americans and Latinos.[18] Later studies repudiated this conclusion.[19] The complexities in analyzing racial variations are seen in the VA study. Biological factors such as variations in drug metabolism may be involved. Other explanations cannot and should not be discounted. The black and Latino men in the study may have been of a lower socioeconomic status than their cohorts. Consequently they would have had more limited access to health care and their health status may have been poorer even before they became HIV positive. In addition, they may have had more advanced disease than their cohorts.

The use of race as a variable in clinical medicine and medical research should continue to be carefully examined. Race is usually used reflexively and without much thought. For example, one of the first things that American medical students learn is to take medical histories. They are usually taught to identify the patient, first and foremost, by age, race, and sex—"This is a thirty-two-year old black female." This identification holds even if a patient is presenting with a sprained ankle. It is not always clear what the patient's race has to do with diagnosis, prognosis, or therapy. Furthermore, it is assumed that a health care provider will know how to "diagnose" race. This, however, is a social skill learned in a race-conscious society, not as a matter of scientific instruction.

The point is not to ignore racial differences or deny the significance of race as a variable in medical research. Rather it is to urge researchers to make clear what they measuring and in what ways they are using the term "race." As social scientists Doris Wilkinson and Gary King have argued:

> Health researchers who employ race as an empirical variable must understand the environmental context in which this ambiguous and value-laden concept thrives. They have a responsibility to define its meaning and theoretical applications with greater precision than has heretofore been the case. As scientists, they also have an obligation to assess objectively and predict the social and economic ramifications of using race in a particular way.[20]

Their words serve to remind us that health policy initiatives and research agendas will differ according to what definition of race is employed. These divergent interpretations of race raise profound questions about what is being measured when racial differentials in research are ascertained. Are the effects of physiological or anatomical differences being measured? Are the effects of genetic differences being measured? Are the effects of the lack of adequate health care being measured? Are the effects of racism being measured? Are the effects of socioeconomic status *and* genetic endowment being measured? These are questions that must be addressed as programs are developed to include more women of color in research programs. The many unanswered questions regarding racial differences in medical research mandates more precision in the use of the term and the development of strategies to include more people of color in clinical studies.

The Dangers of Difference in Medical Research

In a recent article, law professor Patricia A. King warned that medical researchers have to be careful when they analyze racial differences between blacks and whites. She writes, "In a racist society that incorporates beliefs about the inherent inferiority of African American in contrast to the superior status of whites, any attention to the question of differences that may exist is likely to be pursued in a manner that burdens rather than benefits African Americans."[21] King's comments underscore the dangers of difference in medical research. Medicine does not operate in a vacuum. It has reflected and reinforced the beliefs and values of the wider society. Accordingly, it has been influenced by issues of race and racism. History shows numerous examples of the use of medical thought to support the political ideology that black people are inferior. Medical theories, for example, were used to justify the enslavement of Africans. An analysis of the theories behind the decline in the fertility rates of black women between 1880 and 1940 illustrates this danger of difference. It demonstrates how biological and medical arguments have been used to reinforce and perpetuate stereotypes about black women. It also shows how biological explanations have overridden alternative hypotheses. The fertility rate for white women also dropped, but not to the same degree. However, the theories explaining a similar phenomenon in the two groups varied. The explanations were viewed through the prism of race.

The traditional view has been to attribute the decline in the fertility rate among black women to biological and medical factors, including venereal disease, puerperal septicemia, rickets, pellagra, and tuberculosis.[22] The dominant paradigm to explain the differentials, the so-called "health hypothesis", specifically points to a high rate of venereal disease in black women as the major factor behind the numbers. An alternative explanation, however, was offered to explain the concurrent trend in white women. White women, it was argued, used contraceptive measures such as abstinence, barrier methods, rhythm, and withdrawal. The decline in the African American rate was portrayed as involuntary, while the white rate as voluntary.

Many physicians and social scientists believed that low intelligence and high immorality among black women prevented their use of contraception. In 1932 Raymond Pearl, one of the major proponents of the health hypothesis, alleged that black women's contraceptive use was lower than that of their white counterparts because "the negro generally exercises less prudence and foresight than white people do in all sexual matters."[23] The authors of a 1958 book on childbirth and abortion also emphasized the perceived racial differences in reproductive behavior. They wrote:

> Insofar as reproductive behavior is concerned, the . . . pattern [for most blacks] may be simply described as inevitable, natural, and desirable activity to be enjoyed both in and out of marriage; contraception is little known and considered at best a nuisance and at worst dangerous or unnatural; and pregnancy is accepted as an inevitable part of life.[24]

The perception of black women as less willing and less able to control their fertility continues to haunt as today, most notably in the debates surrounding the use of Norplant and Depo-Provera.[25]

The health hypothesis achieved its dominant position, in part, because it fit stereotypical notions about the alleged promiscuity of black women. Roger Lane in his 1986 award-winning book, *The Roots of Violence in Black Philadelphia, 1860–1900,* suggests that prostitution and venereal disease significantly impaired the fertility of black women at the turn of the century. He writes, "All told, perhaps a quarter of Philadelphia's black women who reached the end of their childbearing years had at some time had exposure to the diseases and habits associated with prostitution. This figure would certainly account almost precisely for the difference between black and white fertility in the city."[26] Stereotypical ideas about black women were even incorporated into medical textbooks. In the early 1970s *Novak's Textbook of Gynecology* proclaimed, "Currently, it would appear that the newer antibiotics may completely cure salpingitis without the usual residue of "closed tubes" and sterility. Unquestionably, this is a factor in the increased Negro birth rate."[27]

In recent years, the validity of the health hypothesis has been challenged and substitute explanations have been put forth to explain the decline in the fertility rates of black women. Proponents of these alternate theories argue that biological factors, especially the chronic poor health of black women, may have played a role, but that other socioeconomic considerations must not be discounted. Close historical examination of the lives of African American women reveals images that sharply contrast to the previously accepted view. Jessie Rodrique has discovered that a nationwide, grass roots birth control movement operated in the black community in the years before World War II. An analysis of this movement clearly demonstrates that black women and men used contraceptive methods.[28] Additional studies, including those of social scientists Joseph A. McFalls and George S. Masnick, support this contention. McFalls and Masnick conducted extensive interviews with black women and found that they had used a broad range of contraceptive measures throughout the twentieth century. The researchers concluded:

> The three propositions usually advanced to support the view that birth control had little, if any, effect on black fertility from 1880 to 1940—that blacks used 'ineffective' methods, that blacks did not practice birth control 'effectively,' and that blacks used birth control too late in their reproductive careers to have had much of an effect on their fertility—simply have no empirical or even a priori foundation. There is no reason now to believe that birth control had little impact on black fertility during this period.[29]

Darlene Clark Hine argues that African American women who migrated to northern cities often practiced abstinence to gain economic security and personal autonomy.[30] She also points out how racism and sexism influenced previous studies. She writes, "Only latent acceptance of the myths concerning the alleged unbridled passions and animalistic sexuality of black women prevent serious consideration of the reality and extent of self-determined celibacy." It should also be noted that the health hypothesis ignored issues of class. Middle-class women, regardless of race, had fewer children than poor and working class women. This points to an inconsistency in the hypothesis—black women "with the socioeconomic and educational characteristics most conducive to good health had the lowest fertility and the highest childlessness."[31] The current consensus is that many factors appear to have influenced the fertility rates of African American women from 1880 to 1840.

The history of the theories surrounding these rates show some of the dangers involved in explaining racial differentials. The fecundity of both black and white women declined during the period. However, different interpretations were often sought to explain the event in the two racial groups. Racism frequently shaped these interpretations. The health hypothesis, a theory that reflected and reinforced stereotypical notions of African American women, was the predominant paradigm for many years. In addition, once again we see how a tendency toward biological explanations may obscure the significance of socioeconomic factors.

The myth of racial immunity is another dilemma that can result from an overemphasis on race as an independent variable in medical research and clinical medicine. The implications of this myth are clearly demonstrated in studies of race and osteoporosis. The 1984 National Institutes of Health (NIH) Consensus Development Conference Statement on Osteoporosis called the bone disorder a major public health problem.[32] Researchers estimate that one-third of all women between the ages of 45 and 75 will develop osteoporosis. In concert with traditional public health practices, physicians and researchers have focused on identifying risk factors and developing intervention strategies. The NIH statement classified white women as the most at risk population. Black women, it noted, developed the condition much less frequently. In the years since the release of the NIH statement, campaigns to prevent the bone disorder have focused primarily on white women.

Age and gender are the primary risk factors for osteoporosis. However, studies have also stressed the importance of race and ethnicity. Osteoporosis is often portrayed as "a unique phenomenon of relatively inactive, postmenopausal, white females, fragile in outer appearance, and given to little consumption of milk or other dairy products."[33]

Women of color are frequently pictured as being relatively immune to the condition. One 1987 review went so far as to declare, "It is a well-known fact that blacks do not suffer from osteoporosis."[34] The low incidence of osteoporosis in African American women has been attributed to biological factors including increased bone mass and decreased bone resorption.[35] These studies have failed, however, to control for other factors known to affect bone density, such as weight, diet, health, alcohol intake, cigarette smoking, exercise level, and reproductive history. Race is also seen in these investigations as a definable genetic category.

Additional studies have concluded that Hispanic women are also less susceptible to the disorder than white women.[36] One author has suggested that as Mexican Americans and African Americans are "relatively protected" that they "may benefit less from prophylactic theories."[37] The literature on Asians is contradictory with studies presenting them as both less and more susceptible.[38] Race and ethnicity, however, do not offer immunity to osteoporosis. Black and Hispanic women do get the disease, albeit at lower rates than white women. Less susceptible is not equivalent to immune.

Targeting susceptible populations for screening and educational programs is a well-established public health practice. However, we must be careful not to allow confused notions of racial susceptibility to influence inappropriately public health policy and the practice of medicine. Factors other than race play roles in the divergent incidences of osteoporosis in black and white women. Race must not be used as the dominant risk factor. We must evaluate each woman on an individual basis and assess other risk factors. An examination of race and osteoporosis suggests the danger of using race to define a disease. Osteoporosis is not a white woman's disease. However, most prevention and screening programs have been directed toward them. The question remains as to what extent the myth of racial immunity has led to unwarranted neglect of the health care needs of women of color.

A Legacy of Distrust: A Research Obstacle

Although recent studies have criticized the underrepresentation of women in clinical studies, it is important to know that poor and minority women have, at times, been exploited in the name of science and medicine. An understanding of this past history will demonstrate why so many people of color are mistrustful of the medical profession and its institutions. As efforts begin to include more women of color in clinical research, it is imperative that this legacy of distrust be addressed and not be dismissed as paranoia or hypersensitivity. The challenge before us is to attempt to understand and confront the historically based realities behind these sentiments.

The Tuskegee Syphilis Study symbolizes for many African Americans the racism that pervades American institutions, including the medical profession.[39] It is often used to demonstrate why African Americans should not cooperate with medical researchers. The United States Public Health Service (USPHS) initiated the study in 1932 in order to document the natural history of syphilis. The subjects of the investigation were 400 poor black sharecroppers from Macon County, Alabama, with latent syphilis and 200 men without the disease who served as controls. The physicians conducting the study deceived the men, telling them they were being treated for "bad blood." For example, the men were informed that lumbar punctures were therapeutic, not diagnostic.

As part of the project, however, the USPHS deliberately denied treatment to the men who had syphilis and went to extreme lengths to ensure that they would not receive any. When the Tuskegee Syphilis study began, the standard therapy for syphilis consisted of painful injections of heavy metal compounds such as arsenic and bismuth which had to be administered for up to two years. Although this therapy was less effective than penicillin would later prove to be, in the 1930s every major textbook on syphilis recommended it for the treatment of the disease at all stages. Published medical reports have estimated that between 28 and 100 men died as a result of their syphilis. In exchange for their participation the men received free meals, free medical examinations, and burial insurance.

The Tuskegee Syphilis Study continued until 1972. Throughout its 40 year history, accounts of the study appeared in prominent medical journals. Thus, the experiment was widely known in medical circles. As late as 1969, a committee from the Centers for Disease Control examined the study and decided to continue it. Three years later, a USPHS worker, who was not a physician, leaked details about it to the press. Media disclosure and the subsequent public outrage led to the termination of the study and ultimately to the National Research Act of 1974. This act, established to protect subjects in human experimentation, mandates institutional review board (IRB) approval of all federally funded research using human subjects.

The Tuskegee Syphilis Study raises questions not only about human experimentation, but also about racism in medicine. White physicians in the late nineteenth and early twentieth centuries wrote extensively about the health problems of African Americans, especially syphilis. They maintained that intrinsic racial characteristics such as excessive sexual desire, immorality, overindulgence, and anatomical differences—large penises and small brains—caused black people to have high rates of syphilis. The physicians also believed that syphilis was difficult to treat in black patients because they could not be convinced to come in for treatment or, if they did, to follow the treatment regimen.

Historian Allan Brandt has argued that these assumptions regarding black people and venereal disease influenced the physicians who initiated the Tuskegee Syphilis Study. He writes, "The premise that blacks, promiscuous and lustful, would not seek or continue treatment, shaped the study. A test of untreated syphilis seemed 'natural' because the USPHS presumed the men would never be treated; the Tuskegee Study made that a self-fulfilling prophecy."[40]

The Tuskegee Syphilis Study did not occur in a vacuum. It represented the continuing influence of racist thought not only on medical theory, but on physicians' perceptions of a group of people and consequently on the treatment—or lack of treatment—individuals would receive.

After the Study had been exposed, many black people charged that it represented "nothing less than an official, premeditated policy of genocide."[41] Most recently, both genocide and Tuskegee have come up with respect to AIDS. In September 1990, an article entitled "Is It Genocide?" appeared in *Essence,* a black woman's magazine. The author noted, "As an increasing number of African-Americans continue to sicken and die and as no cure for AIDS has been found some of us are beginning to think the unthinkable: Could AIDS be a virus that was manufactured to erase large numbers of us? Are they trying to kill us with this disease?"[42] In other words, some members of the black community see

AIDS as part of a deliberate plot to exterminate African Americans. Although there is not any credible scientific evidence to support such claims, these ideas should not be dismissed as being merely those of paranoid extremists. For example, a 1990 survey conducted by the Southern Christian Leadership Conference found that 35 percent of the 1,056 black church members who responded believed that AIDS was a form of genocide.[43] The Tuskegee Syphilis Study is presented as evidence of the government's genocidal policies toward African Americans.

A lasting legacy of the study is that it demonstrates to many African Americans why they should not trust the medical profession. Dr. Stephen B. Thomas, co-director of the Minority Health Research Laboratory at the University of Maryland College Park, laments, "Although everyone may not know the *specifics* of the Tuskegee experiment, they have enough residual knowledge of it so that they mistrust government-sponsored programs, and this results in a lack of participation in [AIDS] risk-reduction efforts."[44]   Alpha Thomas, a health educator at Dallas's University Hospital, often confronts the legacy of Tuskegee. She notes that "so many African American people that I work with do not trust hospitals or any of the other community health care service providers because of that Tuskegee Experiment. It is like . . . if they did it then they will do it again."[45]

These apprehensions contribute to the low enrollment rate of African-Americans in clinical trials.[46]   A 1989 study conducted by pharmacologist Craig K. Svensson demonstrated the underrepresentation of African Americans in clinical trials He reviewed 50 clinical trials for new drugs that had been published in *Clinical Pharmacology and Therapeutics* for the three year period 1984–1986. He discovered that the proportion of black subjects was less than their percentage in the cities in which the research was conducted and less than their percentage in the general population of the United States. More recent studies confirm this underrepresentation of African-Americans in clinical trials for AIDS drugs.[47]

The strengthening of safeguards and the reforms in research standards that followed the public disclosure of the abuses of the Tuskegee Syphilis Study, have been insufficient to change African Americans' historically based fears of medical research. The tenacity of this conviction is understandable if one examines the broader history of race and American medicine. The historical record makes clear that although the Tuskegee Syphilis Study may have been an extreme example, it was not an isolated aberration. It was not the only case in the history of medicine where people of color have been exploited in the name of medicine.

The foundation of modern gynecology, for example, is based on the sacrifices of three slave women. Between 1845 and 1849 Dr. J. Marion Sims, the so-called father of modern gynecology, used the women as subjects of experiments designed to develop an operative technique to repair vesico-vaginal fistulas. The three slave women on whom Sims operated each underwent up to 30 painful operations. The physician himself described the brutality of some of his experiments. He wrote, "The first patient I operated on was Lucy. . . . That was before the days of anesthetics, and the poor girl, on her knees, bore the operation with great heroism and bravery."[48] This operation was not successful and Sims later attempted to repair the defect by placing a sponge in the bladder. This experiment, too, ended in failure. He noted, "The whole urethra and the neck of the bladder were in a high state of inflammation, which came from the foreign substance. It had to come away, and there was nothing to do but to pull it away by main force. Lucy's agony was extreme. She was much prostrated, and I thought that she was going to die; but by irrigating the parts of the bladder she recovered with great rapidity. . . ."[49] Sims finally did perfect his technique and ultimately repaired the fistulas. Only after his experimentation with the slave women proved successful did the physician attempt the procedure on white women volunteers. He found, however, that they could not, or more accurately, would not, withstand the pain and discomfort that the procedure entailed. The black women had no choice but to endure. They were forced to submit because the state considered them property and denied them the legal right to refuse to participate.

Abuse of women of color by the medical profession extended into the twentieth century. Some of the most predominant examples have revolved around contraception. In one study conducted in 1969 at a family planning clinic in Austin, Texas poor women, mostly Chicanas, received what they believed to be contraceptives.[50] However, 76 patients, without their knowledge, received placebos. Those who became pregnant were not provided with abortion services even after they requested it. In the 1970s numerous reports of sterilization abuses against women of color surfaced.[51] In the 1974 Relf case, a federal district court found that an estimated 100,000 to 150,000 poor women were sterilized annually under federally funded programs. Some of these women had been coerced into consenting to the procedure by threats that failure to do so would result in the termination of welfare payments.

History, however, is not just about the past. It profoundly affects our contemporary lives. A historically based legacy of distrust still influences the relationship of people of color to the medical profession. It is a significant obstacle to the initiatives to include more women of color in clinical research. One of the challenges that the profession faces is to not to dismiss this sentiment, but to confront it and change it. Efforts should be made to find out what women of color need and want from the health care system. Researchers associated with a new research project at the Centers for Disease Control and Prevention have acknowledged that the voices and experiences of African American women are crucial for the project's success. This investigation is designed to analyze the impact of psychosocial factors on the incidence of preterm delivery among black women. In a radical departure from traditional scientific studies, the investigators have actively solicited advice about the study from the African American lay community. Their goal is to develop a collaborative research strategy that is viewed as a study that is done with black women, not on them.[52,53]

Recommendations

It is not inappropriate to take race into account when clinical research programs involving women are developed. However, the use of race as a variable must be used cautiously and judiciously. History has shown that racial differences have been frequently used without precision. Investigators should make clear how race is being defined in their studies. They should also delineate what they are measuring in research designed to analyze racial differences. Are they using race as a proxy for physiological differences, socioeconomic status, inadequate access to health care? Researchers should also make clear what factors prompted them to explore racial differences. Was it based on observations? Or on preconceived notions that differences should exist? Or on past experiments that did not control for other risk factors? Or on stereotypes about racial minorities? History has also demonstrated that research on racial differences has at times had detrimental effects on people of color. We cannot allow racist and sexist notions about groups of people to influence clinical studies. Finally, programs must be implemented to confront the distrust that people of color have toward the medical profession. The development of collaborative research strategies as proposed by the CDC study of preterm deliveries is a much-needed step.

NOTES

1. Evelyn Brooks Higginbotham, "African-American Women's History and the Metalanguage of Race," *Signs* 17 (1992): 253.

2. Ibid.

3. For more extensive examinations of the history of racial classification,see Nancy D. Fortney, "The Anthropological Concept of Race," *Journal of Black Studies* 8 (September 1977): 35–54; Ashley Montague, ed., *The Concept of Race* (Glencoe, IL: Free Press, 1964).

4. F. James Davis, *Who is Black?: One Nation's Definition* (University Park: Pennsylvania State University Press, 1991); Barbara Jean Fields, "Slavery, Race, and Ideology in the United States of America," *New Left Review* 181 (1990): 95–118; Richard Graham, ed., *The Idea of Race in Latin America* (Austin: University of Texas Press, 1990); Christopher S. Wren, "South Africa Scraps Law Defining People By Race," *New York Times*, 18 June 1991.

5. Robert A. Hahn, "The State of Federal Health Statistics on Racial and Ethnic Groups," *JAMA* 267 (1992):268–71.

6. Cited in Elazar Barkar, *The Retreat of Scientific Racism: Changing Concepts of Race in Britain and the United States Between the World Wars* (Cambridge: Cambridge University Press), p. 341.

7. Richard C. Lewontin, Steven Rose, and Leon J. Kamin, *Not in Our Genes: Biology, Ideology, and Human Nature* (New York: Pantheon, 1984), p. 127.

8. George Stocking, *Race, Culture, and Evolution: Essays in the History of Anthropology* (New York: Free Press, 1968), p. 163.

9. Fatimah Linda Collier Jackson, "Race and Ethnicity as Biological Constructs," *Ethnicity and Health* 2 (Spring 1992): 122–123.

10. Richard Cooper, "A Note on the Biologic Concept of Race and Its Application in Epidemiological Research," *American Heart Journal* 108 (1984): 722.

11. Richard Cooper, "The Biological Concept of Race and Its Application to Public Health and Epidemiology," *Journal of Health Politics, Policy, and Law* 11 (1986): 97–116; Vicente Navarro, "Race or Class Versus Race and Class: Mortality Differentials in the United States," *Lancet* 336 (1990): 1238–1240.

12. Vicente Navarro, "The Class Gap," *The Nation*, 8 April 1991, p. 436.

13. Richard Cooper, "A Note on the Biologic Concept of Race," p. 716.

14. Newton G. Osborne and Marvin D. Feit, "The Use of Race in Medical Research," *JAMA* 267 (1992): 275.

15. Keith Wailoo, "A Disease Sui Generis: The Origins of Sickle Cell Anemia and the Emergence of Modern Clinical Research, 1904–1924," *Bulletin of the History of Medicine* 65 (1991): 185–208.

16. See Warren E. Leary, "Sickle-Cell Screening Urged for All Newborns," *New York Times,* 28 April 1993.

17. For an overview of the topic, see Richard A. Levy, *Ethnic and Racial Differences in Response to Medicines* (Reston, VA: National Pharmaceutical Council, 1993).

18. Paul Cotton, "Race Joins Host of Unanswered Questions on Early HIV Therapy," *JAMA* 265 (1991): 1065–1066.

19. S. Langakos et. al., "Effects of Zidovudine Therapy in Minority and Other Subpopulations with Early HIV infection," *JAMA* 266 (1991): 2709–2712; P.J. Easterbrook, "Racial and Ethnic Differences in Outcome in Zidovudine-treated Patients with Advanced HIV Disease," *JAMA* 266 (1991): 2713–2718.

20. Doris Y. Wilkinson and Gary King, "Conceptual and Methodological Issues in the Use of Race as a Variable: Policy Implications," in *Health Policies and Black Americans,* ed. David P. Willis (New Brunswick, NJ: Transaction Publishers), p. 68.

21. Patricia A. King, "The Dangers of Difference," *Hastings Center Report* 22, no. 6 (1992): 35.

22. Joseph A. McFalls, Jr., and Marguerite Harvey McFalls, *Disease and Fertility* (New York: Academic Press, 1984); Paul Wright, "An Examination of Factors Influencing Black Fertility Decline in the Mississippi Delta, 1880–1930," *Social Biology;* Reynolds Farley, *Growth of the Black Population: A Study of Demographic Trends* (Chicago: Markham, 1970); P. Cutright and E. Shorter, "The Effects of Health on the Completed Fertility of Nonwhite and White U.S. Women Born Between 1867 and 1935," *Journal*

of Social History 13 (1979): 191–217.

23. Raymond Pearl, "Contraception and Fertility in 2,000 Women," *Human Biology* 4 (1932): 395.

24. P.W. Gebhard, W. Pomeroy, C. Martin, and C. Christenson, *Pregnancy, Birth, and Abortion* (New York: Harper and Brothers, 1958), p. 154 quoted in Joseph A. McFalls, Jr. and George S. Masnick, "Birth Control and the Fertility of the U.S. Black Population, 1880 to 1980," *Journal of Family History* 6 (1981): 104.

25. Felicity Barringer, "Making Birth Control Easier Raises Touchy Political Issues," *New York Times*, 8 November 1992; Alex S. Jones, "Editorial Linking Blacks, Contraceptive Stirs Debate at Philadelphia Paper," *Arizona Daily Star*, 23 December 1990.

26. Roger Lane, *The Roots of Violence in Black Philadelphia, 1860–1900* (Cambridge: Harvard University Press, 1986), p. 159.

27. Cited in Janet L. Mitchell, "Provision of Care for Women: Challenges and Opportunities" (paper presented at the National Conference on Women and HIV Infection, Washington, D.C., 14 December 1990), p. 2.

28. Jessie M. Rodrique, "The Black Community and the Birth Control Movement," in *Passion and Power: Sexuality and History,* ed. Kathy Peiss and Christina Simmons (Philadelphia: Temple University Press, 1989), pp. 138–154.

29. McFalls and Masnick, "Birth Control and the Fertility of the U.S. Black Population," p. 103.

30. Darlene Clark Hine, "Black Migration to the Urban Midwest: The Gender Dimension, 1915–1945," in *The Great Migration in Historical Perspective,* ed. Joe William Trotter, Jr. (Bloomington: Indiana University Press, 1991), pp. 134–137. (See p. 135.)

31. McFalls and Masnick, "Birth Control and the Fertility of the U.S. Black Population," p. 90.

32. J.F. Kelsey, "Osteoporosis: Prevalence and Incidence," *Consensus Development Conference Summary, National Institutes of Health* 5 (April 1984): 25–28.

33. Stanley M. Garn, "Bone-loss and Aging," *Physiology and Pathology of Human Aging* (1975): 1–18.

34. Susan Helene Scherf Wasserman and Uriel S. Barzel, "Osteoporosis: The State of the Art in 1987: A Review," *Seminars in Nuclear Medicine* 17 (1987): 285.

35. Mildred Trotter, "Densities of Bones of White and Negro Skeletons," *Journal of Bone and Joint Surgery* 42 (1960): 50–58; S.H. Cohn et al.; "Comparative Skeletal Mass and Radial Bone Mineral Content in Black and White Women," *Metabolism* 26 (1977): 171–178; Mary E. Farmer et al., "Race and Sex Differences in Hip Fracture Incidence," *American Journal of Public Health* 74 (1984): 1374–1380; Robert S. Weinstein and Norman H. Bell, "Diminished Rates of Bone Formation in Normal Black Adults," *New England Journal of Medicine* 319 (1988): 1688–1701.

36. Richard Bauer and Richard Deyo, "Low Risk of Vertebral Fracture in Mexican American Women," *Archives of Internal Medicine* 147 (1987): 1437–1439; Richard Bauer, "Ethnic Differences in Hip Fracture: A Reduced Incidence in Mexican Americans," *American Journal of Epidemiology* 127 (1988): 145–149.

37. Bauer, "Ethnic Differences," p. 145.

38.   David R. Rudy, "Osteoporosis: Overcoming A Costly and Debilitating Disease," *Postgraduate Medicine* 86 (1989): 151–158; Stuart Silverman and Roberta Madison, "Decreased Incidence of Hip Fracture in Hispanics, Asians, and Blacks: California Hospital Discharge Data," *American Journal of Public Health* 78 (1988).

39.   James H. Jones, *Bad Blood: The Tuskegee Syphilis Experiment,* 2nd ed. (New York: Free Press, 1993); Allan M. Brandt, "Racism and Research: The Case of the Tuskegee Syphilis Study," in *Sickness and Health in America,* 2nd ed., ed. Judith Walzer Leavitt and Ronald L. Numbers (Madison: University of Wisconsin Press, 1985), pp. 331–343.

40.   Allan M. Brandt, "Racism and Research: The Case of the Tuskegee Syphilis Study," in p. 334.

41.   James H. Jones, *Bad Blood* (New York: Free Press, 1981), p. 12.

42.   Karen Grisby Bates, "Is It Genocide?" *Essence,* September 1990, p. 76.

43.   Stephen B. Thomas and Sandra Crouse Quinn, "The Tuskegee Syphilis Study, 1932 to 1972: Implications for HIV Education and AIDS Risk Education Programs in the Black Community," *American Journal of Public Health* 81 (1991): 1499.

44.   Karen Grisby Bates, "Is It Genocide?" *Essence,* September 1990, p. 116.

45.   Cited in Thomas and Quinn, "The Tuskegee Syphilis Study," p. 1503.

46.   Craig K. Svensson, "Representation of American Blacks in Clinical Trials of New Drugs," *JAMA* 261 (1989): 263–265.

47.   Robert Steinbrook, "AIDS Trials Shortchange Minorities and Drug Users," *Los Angeles Times,* 25 September 1989, pp. 1, 19; Mark D. Smith, "Zidovudine: Does It Work For Everyone?", ed., *JAMA,* 266 (1991): 2750–2751.

48.   J. Marion Sims, *The Story of My Life* (New York: Appleton, 1889), pp. 236–237.

49.   *Ibid.,* p. 238.

50.   Aileen Adams and Geoffrey Cown, "The Human Guinea Pig: How We Test New Drugs," *World,* 5 December 1972, p. 21.

51.   Helen Rodriguez-Trias, "Sterilization Abuse," *Women's Health* 3 (May–June 1978): 10–15; *Relf v. Weinberger,* 372 *Federal Supplement* (1974): 1196–1205; Laurie Nsiah-Jefferson, "Reproductive Laws, Women of Color, and Low-Income Women," in *Reproductive Laws, Women of Color, and Low-Income Women,* ed. Sherrill Cohen and Nadine Taub (Clifton, NJ: Humana Press), pp. 23–67.

52.   *Relf v. Weinberger.*

53.   Diane L. Rowley, "Racism, Sexism and Social Class: Implications for Preterm Delivery Among Black Women," Centers for Disease Control and Prevention, unpublished.

Health Status of American Indian and Alaska Native Women

Barbara W. Lex and Janice Racine Norris

Socioculturally distinctive groups exhibit differing behaviors associated with disease and health. Members of a group typically share beliefs about etiologies of diseases and what actions to take in response, or "explanatory models."[1] Accordingly, use of medical facilities must be considered in context.[2] The decision to seek treatment not only reflects cultural, gender, and individual beliefs about etiology, but also is influenced by the meaning of seeking help. Decisions to use conventional medical, mental health, or substance abuse services also may be influenced by the general availability of such services, perceived barriers to treatment, actual access to resources and equity in services, or coercion. Individuals usually choose among several treatment options and evaluate the importance of various monetary and nonmonetary costs of treatment. Furthermore, a patient may not make an individual choice, but may follow family or community preferences, including use of alternative therapies offered by traditional healers.

HISTORICAL FACTORS

In contrast to other ethnic minority groups now encompassed within the United States, American Indians and Alaska Natives are descendants of aboriginal peoples who had been in North America for several thousands of years prior to European contact. Archaeologists, physical anthropologists, linguists, and ethnohistorians continue to accumulate knowledge about dates and paths of migrations, which are presumed to stretch from the northeastern portions of Asia, across the Bering Straits, and into the "New World" of the Western Hemisphere.

Status as the "First Americans" is a matter of considerable pride, and, as indigenous peoples, American Indians and Alaska Natives point to the sophistication and complexity of their societies at the time of European contact. Although some were nomadic hunters and gatherers living in groups of 30 to 100, others were members of more numerous tribal groups of sedentary agriculturalists who tilled fields of domesticated plant foods and had political structures that forged alliances between settlements. Still others were organized into larger and more socially complex groups, with massive ceremonial structures, elaborate artistic motifs, and extensive trade relationships with groups at distances of up to a thousand miles.

EARLY IMPACT OF DISEASE AND A LEGACY OF DISTRUST

All aboriginal societies had healers who aided the sick, and in such a context distinctions between religious practices and health practices, as understood by most white Americans, are a largely artificial dichotomy. However, these traditional ministrations had little effect on the variety of diseases introduced by Europeans. "Old World" diseases included "smallpox, measles, the bubonic plague, cholera, typhoid, pleurisy, scarlet fever, malaria, yellow fever, diphtheria, mumps, and whooping cough, and probably typhus and syphilis." Epidemics were recurrent, and accompanying them were "direct and indirect effects of wars (and genocide), enslavements, removals, and relocations, and the destruction of 'ways of life' and subsistence patterns. . . ."[3] For example, smallpox had a profound impact on mortality in children under age five, fetal loss and infertility in women, and possibly infertility in men.

Depopulation from morbidity and mortality also led to general social disorganization and breakdown in performance of social roles. An epidemic of measles that occurred within the last quarter-century in a South American aboriginal group with no immunity provides a glimpse of deteriorating conditions that occurred in the wake of smallpox (and other) epidemics from the seventeenth to the nineteenth century. Caring for children, obtaining food, tending the sick, and attention to sanitary conditions were sufficiently disrupted to increase morbidity and mortality.[4] Previously healthy women and men were so demoralized that many turned their backs, assumed a fetal position in their sleeping hammocks, and awaited death.

Native people recognized that diseases followed encroachment of Europeans, and most believed that epidemics were spread deliberately. For example, major smallpox epidemics occurred during the mid-nineteenth centuries, when "missionary barrels" containing clothing and blankets formerly used by persons infected by smallpox ("fomites") were sent to needy and unsuspecting remnants of displaced tribes. Between 1829 and 1833 outbreaks of malaria decimated coastal native settlements from Vancouver southward to California and also those located in the Columbia River basin.[5] Other historical factors have promoted mistrust. For example, forced assimilation is a highly sensitive issue. Between 1969 and 1974, 25 to 35 percent of American Indian children were placed in institutions, foster care, or adoptive homes. In 1969, it was reported that 85 percent of Indian children in foster placements were in non-Indian homes. Passage of P.L. 95-608 in 1978 (the Indian Child Welfare Act) now requires placement of children with Indian families through tribal authorities.[6]

Placement in off-reservation boarding schools began in 1879.[7] Both male and female children attended these schools, usually beginning at puberty. Boys were taught to be farmers, girls, to be domestic servants. Use of native languages was discouraged, even during recreation and leisure; all pupils wore uniforms. Garments worn by girls were especially designed to deemphasize feminine characteristics and to protect chastity. No personal adornments were permitted, specifically native crafts and hairstyles. Although young people rebelled against regimentation, these experiences permanently marked their perspectives on Indian–white relations. These affronts to Indian identity are still serious issues.

RESERVATION LIVING CONDITIONS

More than two decades ago a landmark five-year demonstration project disclosed the impact of a comprehensive system of primary care services on a previously underserved remote American Indian community.[8] Located near the center of the Navajo Reservation (about 23,000 square miles), Many Farms had a population of about 2,000 persons, most of whom spoke no English. Typically, matrilineal extended families of about 15 persons ("outfits"), comprising an older woman and her husband, their daughters and sons-in-law, and grandchildren, resided in a harsh environment in isolated, poorly ventilated, one-room wood and mud dwellings with dirt floors ("hogans"). About 20 percent of income came from "welfare" sources, and there was a commodities distribution program. Shepherding, odd jobs, weaving, and silver working were major sources of earnings, which for households were $586.00 per year ($147.00 per person) in the early 1960s. Indigenous curers, or medicine men, received respect and much traditional culture was preserved.

Tuberculosis and other respiratory disorders were common. Rashes and fly-borne infectious diseases, such as enteric diseases and trachoma, were promoted by the lack of latrines and ubiquity of domesticated animals. Trauma and severe burns, typical in rural areas, were frequent. Chronic diseases included congestive heart failure, gall bladder disease, and arthritis.[8] Both the birthrate (4 percent increase per annum, or 45.8 per 1,000) and infant mortality rate (55 percent of deaths occurred in the first year of life) were high, and the median age was 15 years. Thus, Navajos at Many Farms three decades ago exhibited a demographic profile now associated with Third World nations. The closest hospital was 55 miles away, one-half of births occurred at home, and hemorrhagic complication of pregnancy was one of the major health problems of women ages 15 to 44. A handful of public health nurses gave smallpox immunizations in school clinics and otherwise cared for about 10,000 persons dispersed over 4,000 to 5,000 square miles.

Primary care physicians were introduced in 1956. Major acute microbial diseases observed during the five-year experiment were pneumonia, diarrhea, otitis media, measles, and impetigo. Only reduction of tuberculosis transmission, decreased incidence of otitis media, and increased referral for hospitalization were attributable to the experiment. The pneumonia-diarrhea complex (cause of about two-thirds of infant deaths) and trachoma (transmitted from child to child by unwashed hands, towels, and utensils) remained serious health problems.[8] Thus, it appears that Navajos at Many Farms needed the services of sanitarians and public health nurses before they could reach a juncture at which they could develop diseases usually considered to require *medical* treatment.

CONTEMPORARY HEALTH PROBLEMS AND ASSESSMENT OF NEEDS

The 1980 and 1990 Censuses indicate that American Indians and Alaska Natives comprise roughly 1 percent of the U.S. population (about 1.75 million persons).[9] They are heterogeneous in tribal origin, preservation of traditions, and extent of urbanization.[10,11,12] Indians became citizens in 1924. In 1953, in an effort to decrease unemployment and encourage immersion into the American mainstream, the Bureau of Indian Affairs, a federal agency, began the Urban Relocation Program to resettle Indians from geographically dispersed remote reservations. Target cities included Boston, Chicago, Cleveland, Dallas, Minneapolis/St. Paul, New York, and San Francisco, but job training and employment did not always materialize and many had to rely on public assistance. As a result of relocation, however, less than 50 percent of Indian people now reside on independently governed reservations (often in widely separated areas), and there are about 300 autonomous groups in the United States.[10,13] In Alaska, 22 ethnic groups are dispersed in 250 villages, and some reside in or near major cities and towns.[14]

It would be exceedingly difficult to conduct a national survey of health status of American Indians and Alaska Natives. Appropriate authorities from each tribal entity, or "reservation," included in the sample would need to grant permission.[15] To learn about Indian people living in towns or cities, where numbers are comparatively small, an adequate health survey would require local oversampling. Even if these obstacles were overcome, definitions of group membership would arise. Like "minorities" or "ethnic groups," there is disagreement about criteria for inclusion. The Bureau of Indian Affairs counts individuals who meet *legal* definitions for registration on tribal rolls, usually quantified by fraction of "blood," with one-fourth to one-eighth minimum as typical. In other instances, persons elect to be known as "Indian" for individual or social reasons, such as intermarriage. For purposes of the United States Census, *self-identification* as American Indian/Alaska Native is adequate.[12,16] For survey purposes, however, even the concept of "household" might not correspond to usage of this term for other minorities. As a consequence, information about Indian health and mental health status is fragmented and uneven in quality.[17]

Native Americans are not included in the National Health and Nutrition Survey (NHANES) conducted by the National Center for Health Statistics, Centers for Disease Control.[18] Most systematic data collection that exists is drawn from patients served by the Indian Health Service (IHS),[19] which potentially serves about 1.1 million people.[9] Both baseline data and routine monitoring systems are needed to meet federally established health objectives, especially for Healthy People 2000.[18] Gaps and limitations have been recognized, and collaboration has begun among the IHS, other federal agencies, and tribal authorities. The Indian Self-Determination and Education Assistance Act of 1975 (P.L. 93-638) established mechanisms that give federally recognized tribes the freedom and power to plan and implement health, educational, and social services.

The predominant health problems among American Indians and Alaska Natives now stem from behavioral risk factors directly related to injuries and chronic diseases.[20,21] Since 1959, the Sanitation Facilities Construction Program of the IHS has improved housing as well as established safe water supplies and adequate waste disposal facilities.[22] As might be expected, there are still unmet needs for a variety of interventions and health services for Native Americans both on and off of reservations.[19] Common problems for adults include lack of prenatal care, need for access to substance abuse or diabetes treatment, and excess deaths from cigarette smoking and alcohol abuse.[23] Problems for adolescents include lack of access to substance abuse or other mental health treatment; deaths from suicide are especially disturbing.[24,25,26]

Cigarette Smoking

Although cigarette smoking among Native Americans has received comparatively little attention, rates are higher than for whites. In 1989, poor school achievement was linked to cigarette use among 31 percent of Indian youth.[24] A study of 119 youths on reservations in Washington found 72 percent of those under age 12 used smokeless tobacco at least once a week.[27] One study of current use of smokeless tobacco use in adults found rates were highest for Plains Indian men, 15 to 20 percent, in contrast to about 5 percent of white men, increasing the risk of oral cavity cancer. Rates for Indian women ranged between 0 and 2 percent.[21]

There is considerable variation according to geographic region. In California in 1989, 40 percent of all deaths of both sexes were attributable to cigarette smoking, in contrast to 17.8 percent and 12.4 percent of white men and women, respectively.[19] In four regions in 1985 to 1988, current cigarette smoking among Native Americans ranged from 14 to 58 percent of women and 18 to 48 percent of men, in contrast to about 25 percent of both white men and women. Highest rates were found in the Plains region, and a separate study of four Indian communities in Montana during 1987–1989 found current smoking rates of 54.5 percent for women and 50.7 percent for men.[21]

Smoking cessation programs for Indian women are important, since infant mortality attributed to maternal smoking includes both respiratory disease and sudden infant death syndrome (SIDS).[28] Lung cancer mortality rates for Indian women in IHS regional units appear to co-vary with rates of tobacco smoking. Tobacco use also contributes to cardiovascular disease, malignant neoplasms, and cerebrovascular diseases. For cancer mortality, lung cancer is the leading cause of death for women in six out of twelve IHS areas, and exceeds the risk for women in the U.S. general population in four areas. Reduction of tobacco smoking prevalence by 20 percent among American Indians is an objective of Healthy People 2000.[29]

Obesity

Among ethnic groups in the United States, overweight and obesity occur most frequently in American Indians.[30] In 1987, the estimated rates of overweight for adult U.S. males and females were 24.1 percent and 25.0 percent, respectively. Rates for American Indian men, 33.7 percent, and women, 40.3 percent, were considerably higher. Among Indian children and adolescents, 24.5 percent of boys and 25 percent of girls were overweight and 11.1 percent of boys and 7.3 percent of girls were obese. For children four years old and under, 11.2 percent were obese (compared to 8.1 percent of U.S. preschool children), with the highest rate for one-year-olds.

An ethnographic study of daily dietary intake of 107 Navajo women found 63 percent to be 20 percent overweight.[31] Subjects had a mean age of 47 years, had attended school for a mean of six years, and most resided about six miles from a food store. Diets were high in saturated fat and refined carbohydrates and low in fiber and vitamin A. Women who were younger and better educated, planted home gardens, read newspapers, had better housing, lived nearer food stores, and had spent more time off of the reservation had better diets.

Household income correlated significantly with dietary intake.

Another ethnographic study compared diets of obese and nonobese Hualapai women in Arizona.[32] Obese women weighed 20 percent or more than desirable weight for height. Subjects were matched for age and percentage of Hualapai ancestry, and were similar in education, income, household composition, marital status, and employment history. Consumption of fat, fiber, and protein did not differ between obese and nonobese women, but obese women consumed more carbohydrates in the form of sweetened soft drinks and alcoholic beverages.

High prevalence of obesity in American Indians is related to hypertension, diabetes, coronary artery disease, poor survival rates for breast cancer, increased rates of gallstones, and poor pregnancy outcome.[33] Prevalence of obesity has surged within the last half-century,[30] and some portion is attributable to the nutritional content of commodity foods distributed to American Indians through feeding programs.[33] Other factors include increased employment among women, the availability of refined carbohydrates from convenience stores and fast food restaurants, and sedentary lifestyle.[32,33] Among Indians, dietary changes may interact with genetic factors,[34] conserving body fat to protect against food shortages.

Diabetes

Diet and physical activity are important throughout the life cycle. Information available about the prevalence of diabetes mellitus (Type 2 diabetes) among Native Americans shows links with obesity, hypertension, anemia, and nutrient deficiencies.[35,36,37] One-third of outpatient visits to the IHS in 1989 were related to diabetes.[38] A recent study of 415 Navajos with Type 2 diabetes[39] found a ratio of females to males of 1.35 to 1, although clinical findings were remarkably similar for women and men. Both weight reduction and increased exercise are involved in treatment of this chronic disease, although many Indian people are found noncompliant with their treatment regimens.

Major studies have focused on the complex interconnection among diet, obesity, diabetes, and pregnancy in Southwestern Indians, especially the Pima tribe. Both genetic and environmental factors are implicated.[40,41] Longitudinal studies have shown that Pima adults currently weigh more than at the turn of the century, and that young adults weigh more than their elders. Higher body mass index predicts risk for Type 2 diabetes, which is familial and associated with lower metabolism, and affects about one-half of the Pima people. However, gestational diabetes mellitus is widespread among Native American women and can lead to higher birthweight babies as well as to Type 2 diabetes in mothers.[42]

In a regional study of behavioral risk factors, about 25 to 35 percent of Native American women (and 25 to 30 percent of Native American men) were found to be overweight (body mass index higher than 27.3 in women and 27.8

in men), in contrast to about 16 to 20 percent of white women and 16 to 23 percent of white men.[21] Sedentary lifestyle (less than three 20-minute sessions of leisure time physical activity per week) was reported by about 40 to 65 percent of Native American women and 44 to 60 percent of Native American men, and 50 to 60 percent of white men and women.[21] In 1989, one study reported that poor health status was linked to overweight and to poor body image among 65 percent of Indian youth.[21]

A follow-up study of 1,012 diabetic male and female Native Americans in Oklahoma examined mortality rates and causes of death.[43] The cohort consisted of 379 men and 633 women diagnosed with non-insulin-dependent diabetes mellitus at baseline during the period 1972-1980. Follow–up was conducted between 1986 and 1989. At that time, 45 percent (452 persons) were deceased, of whom 59 percent were female. Death certificates were obtained and ICD-9 codes analyzed. Major causes of death recorded for the 257 women were circulatory diseases (67 percent), diabetes (26 percent), malignant neoplasms (12 percent), digestive disease (10 percent), and renal disease (6 percent). There was a linear pattern of increased death rates at younger ages, and the ratio of observed to expected deaths for Indian women versus other Oklahoma women was 4.09.

Reproductive Health

Sexually transmitted diseases are associated with complications of pregnancy. One study tested 968 pregnant Navajo women for *Mycoplasma hominis* and *Chlamydia trachomatis* and pregnancy outcome.[44] Half of the women (50 percent) had *M. hominis* and 22 percent, *C. trachomatis.* Complications of pregnancy included 21 percent with preclampsia, 12 percent with postpartum fever or endometritis, and 8 percent with premature rupture of membranes. Sociocultural assessments rated women for "traditionality" (measured by participation in traditional religion, having undergone a Navaho puberty ceremony, or planning a "Blessing Way" ceremony for the baby). *M. hominis* combined with a traditional lifestyle strongly predicted postpartum fever, endometritis, and premature rupture of membranes. It was concluded that "traditionality" could reflect absence of modern conveniences and sanitation or indicate a state of psychological stress associated with the impact of "cultural change."

Another study found rates of *C. trachomatis* among 183 pregnant Indian women to be about 25 percent.[45] Since perinatal infection can cause inclusion conjunctivitis and pneumonia in newborns, prenatal screening of mothers is encouraged. Further, in this population, *Trichomonas* tended to be associated with *C. trachomatis* infection. However, cervical HPV infection rates for

American Indian women appear lower than for Hispanics and non-Hispanic white women.[46]

There is limited information about HIV infection and AIDS prevalence in Indian women.[47] In 1991, 14 percent of 292 American Indian adult and adolescent AIDS cases known to the CDC were female.[48] Risk factors include intravenous drug use, multiple sex partners, early sexual activity, and alcohol use. Perinatally transmitted AIDS affected eight children under age five.[49] In a sample of 481 Indian women in Idaho, Oregon, and Washington,[48] 6.4 percent were at high risk from intravenous drug use, and 30 percent were in the middle group of persons who had sexual intercourse with two or more partners in the previous year. The greatest proportion of high and middle risk women were ages 12 to 29, and 18 to 49, respectively. Middle risk subjects had begun sexual activity at earlier ages and were younger at first pregnancy. They also reported having sexual partners who resided both on and off reservations, which could facilitate transmission of HIV infection from urban to rural areas, and encourage spread of HIV into small communities.

The IHS conducted an HIV seroprevalence survey for the period July 1, 1989, to June 30, 1991.[49] Sources were 37,681 blood specimens obtained from persons being evaluated for STD, entering drug and alcohol treatment programs, or receiving prenatal care in the first or third trimester. One per 3,500 initial prenatal patients and one per 1,000 third trimester/perinatal patients were HIV-1 positive. The rate of HIV-1 infection among patients evaluated for STD was one per 220 males and one per 1,400 females. It was estimated that about 2,300 (range 1,030 to 3,615) men and about 400 (range 180 to 640) women were infected with HIV. During 1990, about 35 infants would have been born to mothers infected with HIV, and, of these, approximately 11 infants would have been infected perinatally.

Fetal alcohol syndrome (FAS) and Fetal Alcohol Effects (FAE) have an impact on Native American infants. May found the lowest FAS rates (1.3 per 1,000) occurred for Navajo women.[50] A much higher rate occurred among Plains Indian women (10.3 per 1,000), and 25 percent of all Plains women with one FAS child also gave birth to others.[50] These findings have prompted local-level studies in other regions.

A behavioral risk factor study was conducted at Warm Springs in Oregon in 1990 among persons over age 18.[22] Of the 234 women surveyed in this study, a pattern of binge drinking was most typical. Among these women, 60 percent reported blackouts, 42 percent had been arrested for driving under the influence of alcohol, 39 percent had received detoxification treatment, and 25 percent had been enrolled in alcohol treatment at least once. In addition, 31 percent had consumed alcohol during their last pregnancy. From a survey of 429 children who had been younger than age 5 on September 1, 1991, 121 were referred for screening for FAS/FAE because of suspected prenatal alcohol exposure, birthweight less than 3,000 grams, or developmental delay. From this sample,

23 were found to meet two criteria, and 19 were evaluated. A total of eight children, four with FAS and four with FAE, were identified. All mothers were over age 30 and had consumed alcohol during pregnancy (there was no assessment of cigarette smoking, inhalant use, or cocaine use). One mother had two children with FAS. A total of seven of the eight children were in foster placement when assessed. Another comprehensive program targeted 48 high-risk Navajo women, of whom 81 percent participated.[51] This program provided alcohol detoxification and family planning services and was hospital based and family oriented, characteristics that seem to have encouraged participation.

During the 1970s, sterilization procedures were performed on poor minority women (black, Hispanic, and Native American).[52] A General Accounting Office (GAO) investigation has examined allegations of genocide by the Bureau of Indian Affairs and the IHS. In a sample of four out of 12 IHS service areas, 3,406 Native American women were found to have been sterilized during 1973–1976. Of these women, 88.1 percent (3,001) were ages 15 to 44.

The IHS now uses protocols to protect patients' rights for both sterilizations,[53] and for the depot contraceptive Norplant.[53,54,55] Sterilization procedures must be voluntary and accompanied by thorough counseling about risks, benefits, and details of the procedure, as well as information about alternative methods of contraception. Only tubal ligation and vasectomy are acceptable, and hysterectomy is prohibited for purposes of sterilization. Sterilization is prohibited for patients under age 21, patients incapable of giving informed consent (i.e., mentally incompetent), or patients institutionalized in a correctional or mental health facility. Informed consent must be documented, and rules of the Department of Health and Human Services must be followed. These rules require that consent be obtained 30 days prior to the procedure routinely, or after 72 hours has elapsed in the case of emergency abdominal surgery. Consent for sterilization cannot be obtained when a woman is in labor, seeking to obtain an abortion, or under the influence of alcohol or any other mind-altering substance. Care providers are encouraged to seek informed consent during the second trimester of pregnancy to avoid exceeding a 180 day limitation for any specific informed consent signature.

Norplant, which now has been used by half a million women in nearly 50 countries, has been available to the IHS since January 1991. A Norplant implant costs $365, which is cost effective for long-term contraception. Generally, Norplant candidates are advised that five years is an optimal time period. Interestingly, Norplant is efficacious because it reduces the amount of cervical mucus and increases its viscosity, creating a barrier preventing migration of sperm through the cervix into the uterus. It inhibits growth of the endometrium and in some patients it suppresses ovulation. The mucus barrier is believed to potentially decrease risk of pelvic infectious disease (PID). High priority patients are women with medical conditions for whom pregnancy might endanger health, women who have recently had an abortion, sexually active teenagers with one or more children, sexually active teenagers (with parental consent) who have plans for career or college education, and women in their twenties who are not ready to contemplate permanent sterilization. Its use is contraindicated in women who are pregnant, have undiagnosed abdominal-uterine bleeding, known or possible breast cancer, thrombo-embolic disease, or liver disease. Other contraindications include migraine headaches, severe obesity, or moderate to severe acne. Norplant is inadvisable for women over age 30, since its use may obscure onset of occult endometrial neoplasia. Any woman planning to have children within four years is advised to seek another contraceptive method.

Infant Mortality

Infant mortality rates for American Indians are difficult to calculate. Accurate rates depend on identification as American Indian on both birth and death certificates. Several studies have shown that high rates (about 20 percent in some areas) of misclassification occur when births and deaths occur outside of IHS facilities.[9]

Primary causes of neonatal (first 28 days of life) death are congenital anomalies, respiratory distress syndrome, disorders related to short gestation and low birthweight (less than 2500 grams), SIDS, effects of maternal complications of pregnancy, and infections specific to the perinatal period.[9] Primary causes of infant (29 to 365 days of life) mortality are SIDS, congenital anomalies, respiratory distress syndrome, disorders related to short gestation and low birthweight, and pneumonia and influenza.[9] It has been estimated that SIDS accounts for 40 percent of postneonatal deaths and 25 percent of infant mortality in Native Americans.[56]

Infant mortality and neonatal death rates vary across the IHS service areas, with lowest rates in the southwestern states and highest in the northern plains and northwest states.[9,57] Infant mortality and neonatal death rates in the Southwest were higher in the past, having improved in recent years, and reflect concerted efforts on the part of the IHS to improve outreach efforts to pregnant women.[9,58,59] Special services are provided to young primigravida women,[60] since in 1987, 19 percent of all low-birthweight Indian infants were born to mothers under age 20.[9]

Cancer, Cardiovascular Disease, and Tuberculosis

A meta-analysis of cancer incidence rates in American Indians versus the general population[61] found reduced incidence of cancer at most sites. Decreased incidence was noted for colon, breast, and uterine cancer. However, increased rates of cervical cancer were observed.

Another meta-analysis of cancer incidence in Indian people[62] found women to have elevated rates of cancers of the gallbladder, cervix, and kidney, but decreased rates for cancers of the colon, breast, and uterus, and for lymphomas. Rates of lung cancer and leukemias were similar. Risk for kidney cancer is associated with obesity, cigarette smoking, and occupational exposures. As noted, obesity occurs for more than half of Indian women, and cigarette smoking by Indian women in some regions is more common than among women in the general population. Gallbladder cancer is associated with benign gallbladder disease as well as obesity and parity, and is more prevalent among Indian than white women. The overall lower cancer mortality rate may be influenced by more immediate causes of excess deaths, such as diabetes, accidents, or infectious diseases.

Respiratory diseases that most severely affect Indian mortality are pneumonia, cancer of the lung, chronic obstructive pulmonary disease (COPD), and tuberculosis.[63] For the period 1980–1986, tuberculosis rates for Indian men and women were 2.2 and 1.7 per 100,000 versus 0.9 and 0.4 for the general U.S. population. Pneumonia rates for Indian people were slightly higher, 24.0 for men and 16.1 for women per 100,000, versus 19.1 for men and 17.6 for women per 100,000 for the general U.S. population. Lung cancer rates for Indian males (19.9 per 100,000) and females (8.8 per 100,000) were considerably lower for the general U.S. population (70.6 and 28.8 per 100,000, respectively). From 1980 to 1986, no emphysema deaths were reported for Indian women or men. Overall, Indians had lower COPD rates (115 per 100,000).

In 1990, the incidence of tuberculosis in American Indians was 18.9 per 100,000.[48] Rates had decreased since 1975, when the incidence rate was 48.0 per 100,000, but rates began to rise again in 1989. In 1990, 39.4 percent of cases (*N* = 146) were female, with 74 percent pulmonary and 26 percent extrapulmonary. The number of cases reported for women dropped from 154 in 1989 to 146 in 1990. These rates are not indicative of tuberculosis secondary to AIDS. The goal for Healthy People 2000 is to reduce the incidence rate to 5 per 100,000. Adequate screening, contact tracing, and treatment efforts by the IHS are being mobilized to attain this objective. Rising rates of cardiovascular disease among Native Americans are the focus of the "Strong Heart Study."[64] Risk factor levels were examined for Indian people living in central Arizona, southwestern Oklahoma, and North and South Dakota. The study focuses on persons ages 35 to 74 and includes a mortality survey to estimate death rates from cardiovascular disease, a morbidity study to estimate incidence of initial and recurrent myocardial infarctions and CVAs, and clinical examinations to estimate the prevalence of risk factors. About 1,500 persons at each site are included in the study. Among the three sites 1,209 females and 1,165 males were enrolled in a 35- to 44-year-old cohort, and 2,175 females and 2,096 males were enrolled in a 45- to 74-year-old cohort.

Prevalence of myocardial infarction, as diagnosed by electrocardiogram, was highest in North and South Dakota Sioux, lower in Indians residing in Oklahoma, and lowest among Pima in Arizona. Contributory factors varied among the three locations. Cholesterol levels were lowest among the Pima, who also had the lowest rate of tobacco smokers. Hypertension was high in Oklahoma tribes and the Pima. All groups had high rates of diabetes and of obesity, but rates were highest among the Pima. Interestingly, more than 90 percent of Pima reported "full-blooded" heritage, in contrast to 73 percent of the Oklahoma tribes and less than half of the Sioux.[65]

Mental Health

It is asserted that mental health problems, including depression, anxiety, suicide, and substance abuse, are greater among Native Americans.[66] Contributing factors are said to include violent behaviors, including physical and sexual abuse.[12] Although suicide rates vary by region and tribe, a recent analysis for the Southwest indicates suicide most frequently occurs among young unmarried males.[67] There are no data available for rates of physical or sexual abuse.

In the absence of systematic research in psychiatric epidemiology, localized studies of small samples provide some empirical data.[68] One study assessed co-morbidity of substance abuse disorders and other psychiatric disorders with the SADS-L.[69] Of 104 adult patients in three mental health clinics, 83 percent had major depression, 50 percent had secondary alcoholism, 20 percent had generalized anxiety, and 17 percent abused drugs. A study conducted in 1988 used the SADS-L to conduct a point prevalence survey among 131 men and women residing in a rural village.[70] A total of 46 percent of men versus 18.4 percent of women had a current psychiatric diagnosis, and 82 percent of men and 58 percent of women had a lifetime diagnosis. Men (36.4 percent) had higher current rates of alcohol abuse or dependence than women (7.0 percent), but women had higher rates for affective disorders (10.3 percent versus 4.6 percent). Men also had diagnoses of organic disorders, schizophrenia, PTSD, and personality disorders, but no women met these criteria. In an unpublished study, of 211 urban Indian women, 17.5 percent met DSM-III-R criteria for alcoholism, 22.3 percent for depression, 12.8 percent for anxiety, and 5.2 percent for drug abuse, but only 15.6 percent received inpatient treatment.[71]

There continue to be gaps in assessment and treatment of mental health problems, including limited availability of outpatient mental health treatment, lack of specialized services for adolescents, and insufficient staff.[68] Inpatient services are typically provided at distant locations, and all services, whether for substance abuse or other psychological disorders, are beset with excessive workloads, inadequate staff training, and lack of continuity for case follow-up. IHS and tribal-based substance abuse services often lack ability to serve the needs of persons with concurrent depression or other disorders.

The IHS Alcoholism and Substance Abuse Program served 25,642 persons in FY 91 and an estimated 37,419 in FY 92 (an increase of about 45 percent).[72] In FY 91 there were 5,638 persons treated in inpatient substance abuse programs, and an estimated 6,811 in FY 92 (an increase of about 20 percent). In FY 92, an estimated 200,349 persons received prevention and intervention services. However, no rates for men versus women are available.

Alcohol Consumption

In the absence of cross-sectional survey data, information from tribal groups or enclaves sketch the parameters of this problem. It should be noted, however, that American Indians and Alaska Natives have attracted disproportionate attention because of reputed excessive alcoholism. One observer stated: "Perhaps no other ethnic group has had more written about their drinking behavior than Native Americans."[11]

High rates of both heavy drinking and abstinence occur among American Indians.[11] May[13,73] found that large disparities in consumption rates were claimed for four different reservation groups with reputations for "hard drinking." Compared with the majority of the general U.S. population (67 percent), 52 to 84 percent of all adults on these reservations reported drinking an alcoholic beverage at least once a year. Abstinence was lowest in Ojibwa (16 percent) and Ute (20 percent), followed by Standing Rock Sioux (42 percent), and highest among Navajo (70 percent).

The highest alcohol use occurs among men age 16 to 29, and usually diminishes after age 35 or 40, so that 30 to 50 percent of middle-aged male abstainers are former moderate or heavy drinkers.[13] However, the number of women who drink may be increasing.[11,74] Rural and urban populations also differ. A comparison of 105 Indians of various tribes who lived in Los Angeles with 86 Indians who lived in rural California[75] found that the urban Indians were about three times more likely to drink two or more times daily (16.2 percent versus 5.8 percent). However, about 60 percent of reservations officially prohibit alcohol use, and prohibition prompts persons who wish to purchase alcohol to drive long distances to obtain it and to drink while driving.[13]

The seriousness of alcohol abuse among Native Americans is reflected in rates of alcoholism-related deaths (deaths attributable to alcohol dependence and alcoholic psychoses as well as liver cirrhosis and chronic liver disease specified as alcoholic). In 1987, the death rate for Native Americans was 25.9 per 100,000 in comparison with 6.0 per 100,000 for all Americans.[76] Deaths from auto crashes are threefold higher among Native Americans, and an unknown but substantial proportion are alcohol-related.[77] In one community almost 10 percent of women (and 20 percent of men) acknowledged driving and drinking.[21] In a study of school performance by 13,454 Indian youths in 1989, poor school achievement was linked with weekly-to-daily alcohol abuse among 20 percent of Indian youth.[24]

Alcohol problems appear to be strongly multigenerational among Native Americans.[78] The 1988 National Health Interview Survey (NHIS) consisted of 43,809 interviews with whites, Hispanics, blacks, and Native Americans.[79] One purpose of the study was to oversample blacks, but 141 male and 201 female Native Americans were included. Although 36.1 percent of all men and 38.8 percent of all women reported having an alcoholic first-, second-, or third-degree relative, highest percentages were reported by Native Americans: 46.1 percent of men but 62.8 percent of women.

Biological Alcohol Susceptibility and Stereotyping

Before European contact, few American Indians residing above the Rio Grande River made use of fermented beverages. Beginning in the seventeenth century,[80] accounts of explorers and missionaries recorded impressions of intoxication occurring among people who had no experience with wine, brandy, and later, rum. May succinctly summarizes the emergence of commonplace beliefs about the effects of alcohol on Native Americans.[13] In the twentieth century, beliefs that "Indians can't hold their liquor" were tested in research laboratories.

In the early 1970s, numerous investigators studied hypothesized differences in sensitivity to alcohol and in metabolism of alcohol in various Asian and Native American groups.[81,82,83,84,85,86,87,88,89,90] Findings have been carefully reviewed.[91] A major premise of such studies is that biological differences in alcohol sensitivity and metabolism may in some way affect vulnerability to alcohol use in certain groups.[91,92,93]

One hypothesis is that persons with increased alcohol metabolism experience rapidly decreased intoxication and, in turn, increase their consumption, while decreased consumption occurs among persons with decreased alcohol metabolism that results in more persistent intoxication. Increased sensitivity to alcohol is manifested by facial and body "flushing" (peripheral vasodilatation), increased heart rate, decreased blood pressure, diaphoresis, nausea, headaches, diarrhea, general dysphoria, rapid absorption and elimination of alcohol, and rapid increase in acetaldehyde levels.[75,91] These responses are primarily exaggerations of the peripheral and internal changes usually produced by alcohol. Intolerance to alcohol may somehow confer protection from alcohol abuse.[91] Increased sensitivity to alcohol has been established in Oriental infants and adults.[75,87] According to Leland,[94] the primary social benefit of identification of increased alcohol sensitivity among American Indians would be an established scientific basis for prevention programs.

Nevertheless, evidence for increased alcohol sensitivity in American Indians is equivocal.[91,92,94]   Fenna and colleagues reported slower rates of alcohol metabolism in Canadian Indians and Inuits than in Caucasian controls.[81] Caucasians manifested a significantly faster disappearance rate than the other two groups, but there were no differences in the amounts of alcohol required to produce peak blood levels.   Wolff found increased facial flushing in Cree Indians,[87] and faster rates of alcohol metabolism occurred in Ojibwa Indians than in Chinese and Caucasian subjects.[88]   No differences in alcohol metabolism were found in a study comparing American Indians and Caucasians,[76] but decreased facial flushing occurred in Tarahumara Indians.[89]   Hanna found lower levels of increased alcohol sensitivity in subjects from populations related to Asiatic gene pools, namely Eskimos, American Indians, Hawaiians, Indochinese, and persons of mixed Asian ancestry.[77]

Emerging interest in the genetics of alcoholism has again stimulated investigation of characteristics of Native Americans.   Interest in the DRD2 dopamine receptor genotype prompted investigation among Cheyenne Indian men, since their frequency of the DRD2 marker allele is fourfold that of Caucasians.[95]

Other investigators are examining frequency of alcohol dehydrogenase alleles and family history of alcoholism in Indian men in California.[96] Additional studies by this research group focus on family history of alcoholism and administer a challenge dose of 75 ml/kg ethanol to measure effects on heart rate and blood pressure.[97]   Yet another study examines EEG records of California Indian men with and without a family history of alcoholism in a drug-free state.[98] Studies of Indian women are planned under similar experimental protocols.

Studies of alcohol sensitivity in American Indians and Alaska Natives require rigorous elicitation of pedigrees in order to establish genetic composition of experimental groups as well as to diminish possible effects of individual differences (cf. notes 92, 94).   Careful selection and matching of subjects and controls also are necessary, especially since there are differences in body structure, composition, and weight, as well as nutritional status and drinking patterns,[91] gender differences in body water distribution,[99] and in "first pass" gastric metabolism.[100]

CURRENT HEALTH CARE NEEDS AND
URGENT RECOMMENDATIONS

Few American Indians have been included in National Health Interview Surveys.   There is a definite need to undertake formal studies of prevalence, incidence, and contributory factors of disease among American Indian groups. To date, health status of American Indians served by the Indian Health Service appears best examined through clinical contacts.   However, it also appears important to identify urban areas with large concentrations of Native American peoples in order to conduct appropriate surveys.

1. American Indian and Alaska Native women should be involved in development of methods of contraception. As noted, fertility and infant mortality among American Indians have demographic profiles similar to those of Third World nations. That is, there is both a high birthrate and a high infant mortality rate. In addition, some groups of Native Americans have an excess concentration of infants affected by FAS or FAE. The need for contraception to reduce the high birthrate and its complications, the high infant mortality rate, and transmission of alcohol-induced insult to the fetus is apparent. However, more permanent contraceptive methods are associated with ethical concerns.

2. American Indians and Alaska Natives should be considered at risk for HIV infection and AIDS. In early 1992 an article appeared in the *Journal of the American Medical Association* entitled "The Challenge of Minority Recruitment in Clinical Trials for AIDS."[101] In this article, discussions of minority participation focused on African American and Hispanic patients. No mention was made of American Indians, who also are at risk for AIDS. A recent publication by the IHS indicated that rates of gonorrhea, chlamydia, primary and secondary syphilis, and PID exceeded rates for all races.[102] In one report published shortly after the *JAMA* article,[103] the number of American Indians infected with HIV was about 2,300 males and about 400 females, and there were about 11 infants with perinatal HIV infection. Rates in urban and rural settings were comparable, an unexpected finding. Yet these findings are likely to underestimate prevalence, since American Indians who had sought HIV testing outside of IHS clinics were not included in the report.

3. Models developed by the IHS clinics should be tested for health care delivery in other settings. Given the seriousness of the AIDS epidemic, specific steps should be taken to increase surveillance and increase education and prevention efforts. Accordingly, sexually active patients are assessed for risk of STDs and HIV, while routine syphilis screening has been instituted for all patients presenting with a possible STD or enrolled in drug and alcohol treatment programs.[103] In addition, early treatment, partner notification, and educational and emotional support for those already infected with HIV need to be put in place to prevent transmission to others. Moreover, efforts are under way to prevent racial misclassification of American Indian and Alaska Native persons with HIV infection or AIDS. This is an important concern, given the need for accurate assessments for morbidity and mortality needed for health planning, resource allocation, and deployment of prevention services.

4. Women's voices should be heard. For example, IHS personnel report moral and medical-legal dilemmas associated with alcoholic women. Alcoholic women are at risk for offspring with FAS or FAE. Unfortunately, these same women often cannot reliably use oral contraceptives and have an increased risk for PID if they use an intrauterine contraceptive device. In this instance, ethical concerns and real medical constraints point to the use of Norplant for patients at

high risk for STDs or for adverse neonatal outcome. Nonetheless, the attention to ethical concerns reflects sophistication and awareness that is commendable. What is missing from the picture, however, are case studies of women considering tubal ligation or utilizing Norplant. It also is important to obtain the perspective of severely alcoholic women and their attitudes toward high risk pregnancies and resultant insults to the fetus.

5. Similar strategies are needed to obtain perspectives from women who are cigarette smokers, diabetic, or obese, or have sick children. With the cooperation of tribal authorities, urban health centers, and the IHS, American Indian women's stories and needs can be expressed.

6. There is an almost complete lack of both published literature and basic data concerning incidence and prevalence of domestic violence among American Indians. Not only do shelters, hospitals, and substance abuse treatment centers need to be encouraged to collect data, compile statistics, and publish reports, but Native American women need to be brought into planning for education and prevention strategies that can most effectively deal with what anecdotal evidence shows to be a pressing health problem.

Participation in research protocols can be influenced by the enthusiasm of the participants. It does not seem likely that a push to enroll large numbers of American Indian women would be successful if they could not see benefits to themselves and others. Risk/benefit calculations often disclose that risks to individuals are outweighed by benefits to society. It appears highly important to enlist cooperation of Indian people in both assessment of their needs and planning research that could ameliorate their own health problems. The example of AIDS risk is particularly compelling. Although there are limited studies, it is interesting to note that the HIV infection rate is comparable in urban and rural areas. This suggests transmission that follows movements of individuals between reservations or rural enclaves and cities. Study of American Indians and AIDS risk appears to present unique factors, but the model that could be developed might have strong implications for other geographically mobile populations.

In sum, it seems most appropriate to seek inclusion of women of racial and ethnic groups into research protocols when diseases and disorders of interest are of special concern in their lives. Any risk-benefit analysis should consider whether a disease entity is more prevalent in a specific racial or ethnic population. Oversampling is needed. In the case of Native Americans, their numbers are small but their health problems loom large.

NOTES

1. A. Kleinman, *Patients and Healers in the Context of Culture: An Exploration of the Borderland between Anthropology, Medicine, and Psychiatry.* 1980, Berkeley, CA: University of California Press.

2. B. W. Lex, "Review of alcohol problems in ethnic minority groups," *J. Cons. Clin. Psychol.* 55 (1987): 293–300.

3. R. Thornton, T. Miller, and J. Warren, "American Indian population recovery following smallpox epidemics," *Am. Anthropol.* 93 (1991): 28–45.

4. J. V. Neel, et al., "Notes of the effect of measles and measles vaccine in a virgin-soil population of South American Indians," *Am. J. Epidemiol.* 91 (1970): 418–429.

5. S. F. Cook, "The epidemic of 1830–1833 in California and Oregon," *Univ. Cal. Publ. Am. Arch. and Ethnol.* 43 (1955): 303–326.

6. J. A. Kessel and S. P. Robbins, "The Indian Child Welfare Act: Dilemmas and needs," *Child Welfare* 53 (1984): 225–232.

7. K. T. Lomawaima, "Domesticity in the federal Indian schools: The power of authority over mind and body," *Amer. Ethnol.* 20 (1993): 227–240.

8. W. McDermott, K. W. Deuschle, and C. R. Barnett, "Health care experiment at Many Farms," *Science* 175 (1972): 23–31.

9. E. R. Rhoades, et al., "Mortality of American Indian and Alaska Native infants," *Ann. Rev. Public Health* 13 (1992): 269–285.

10. D. B. Heath, "American Indians and alcohol: Epidemiological and sociological relevance," in *Alcohol Use Among U.S. Ethnic Minorities,* D. Spiegler, et al. 1989, Washington, DC: U.S. Government Printing Office. Pp. 107–222.

11. J. C. Weibel-Orlando, "Pass the bottle, bro': A comparison of urban and rural Indian drinking patterns," in *Alcohol Use Among U.S. Ethnic Minorities,* pp. 269–290.

12. R. Bachman, *Death & Violence on the Reservation: Homicide, Family Violence, and Suicide in American Indian Populations,* 1992, New York: Auburn House.

13. P. A. May, "Alcohol and alcoholism among American Indians: An overview," in *Alcoholism in Minority Populations,* T. D. Watts and R. Wright, Jr. Springfield, IL: Charles C Thomas. Pp. 95–119.

14. D. Kelso and W. Dubay, "Alaskan Natives and alcohol: A sociocultural and epidemiological review," in *Alcohol Use Among U.S. Ethnic Minorities,* pp. 223–238.

15. E. R. Oetting and F. Beauvais, "Epidemiology and correlates of alcohol use among Indian adolescents living on reservations," in *Alcohol Use Among U.S. Ethnic Minorities,* pp. 239–268.

16. D. B. Heath, "Uses and misuses of the concept of ethnicity in alcohol studies: An essay in deconstruction," *Int. J. Addict.* 25 (1990–91): 607–628.

17. W. A. Vega and R. G. Rumbaut, "Ethnic minorities and mental health," *Ann. Rev. Sociol.* 17 (1991): 351–383.

18. E. D. Nobmann, K. Strauss, and J. Proulx, "Monitoring, research, and evaluation initiative of the IHS nutrition and dietetics section," *The Provider* 17 (1992): 85–86.

19. C. A. Beckwith, "A report on a model using state data to describe the health status and health care needs of Native Americans in California," *The Provider* 17 (1992): 102–109.

20. E. R. Rhoades, "The Indian burden of illness and future health interventions," *Public Health Report* 102 (1987): 361–368.

21. J. R. Sugarman, C. W. Warren, and L. Oge, "Using the behavioral risk factor surveillance system to monitor Year 2000 objectives among American Indians," *Public Health Report* 107 (1992): 449–456.

22. L. S. Gaynor, "IHS sanitation facilities construction program," *The Provider* 17 (1992): 217–219.

23. D. Porter, *Native Americans' Nutrition and Diet Related Diseases.* 1987, Washington, DC: The Library of Congress.

24. R. W. Blum, B. Harmon, and L. Harris, "American Indian-Alaska Native youth health," *The Provider* 17 (1992): 137–146.

25. N. W. Van Winkle and P. A. May, "Native American suicide in New Mexico, 1957–1979: A comparative study," *Hum. Org.* 45 (1986): 296–309.

26. P. A. May, "A bibliography on suicide and suicide attempts among American Indians and Alaska Natives," *Omega* 21 (1990): 199–214.

27. S. P. Schinke, et al., "Native youth and smokeless tobacco: Prevalence rates, gender differences, and descriptive characteristics," in *NCI Monograph 8 NIH Publication No. 89-3055,* F. I. Gregoric, editor, 1989, Bethesda, MD: National Cancer Institute. Pp. 39–42.

28. M. Bulterys, et al., "The expected impact of a smoking cessation program for pregnant women on infant mortality among Native Americans," *Am. J. Prev. Med.* 6 (1990): 267–273.

29. B. Leonard, et al., "IHS tobacco project," *The Provider* 18 (1993): 107–116.

30. Brenda A. Broussard, et al., "Prevalence of obesity in American Indians and Alaska Natives," *Am. J. Clin. Nutr.* 53 (1991): 1535S–1542S.

31. W. S. Wolfe and D. Sanjur, "Contemporary diet and body weight of Navajo women receiving food assistance: An ethnographic and nutritional investigation," *J. Am. Diet. Assoc.* 88 (1988): 822–827.

32. N. I. Teufel and D. L. Dufour, "Patterns of food use and nutrient intake of obese and non-obese Hualapai Indian women of Arizona," *J. Am. Diet. Assoc.* 90 (1990): 1229–1235.

33. T. K. Welty, "Health implications of obesity in American Indians and Alaska Natives," *Am. J. Clin. Nutr.* 53 (1991): 1616S–1620S.

34. J. V. Neel, "Diabetes mellitus: A 'thrifty' genotype rendered detrimental by 'progress'?" *Am. J. Hum. Gen.* 14 (1962): 353–362.

35. E. D. Nobmann, T. Byers, and A. P. Lanier, "The diet of Alaska Native adults: 1987–1988," *Am. J. Clin. Nutr.* 55 (1992): 1024–1032.

36. C. Ritenbaugh, "New approaches to old problems: Interactions of culture and nutrition," in *Clinically Applied Anthropology: Anthropologists in Health Science Settings,* N. J. Chrisman and T. W. Maretzki, editors. 1982, Dordrecht, Holland, & Boston, MA: D. Reidel Publishing Company.

37. L. T. Montour, A. C. Macaulay, and N. Adelson, "Diabetes mellitus in Mohawks of Kahnawake, PQ: A clinical and epidemiologic description," *CMAJ* 141 (1989): 549–552.

38. H. A. J. Walden, "Reorganizing diabetes clinics to enhance patient involvement and reduce staff stress," *The Provider* 17 (1992): 92–95.

39. W. Hoy, et al., "Navajo Indians with Type 2 diabetes," *The Provider* 18 (1993): 41–48.

40. B. W. Howard, C. Gogardus, and E. Ravusin, "Studies of the etiology of obesity in Pima Indians," *Am. J. Clin. Nutr.* 53 (1991): 1577S–1585S.

41. W. C. Knowler, D. J. Pettitt, and M. F. Saad, "Obesity in Pima Indians: Its magnitude and relationship with diabetes," *Am. J. Clin. Nutr.* 53 (1991): 1543S–1551S.

42. N. B. Attico, K. C. Smith, and A. G. Waxman, "Diabetes mellitus in pregnancy: Views toward an improved perinatal outcome," *The Provider* 17 (1992): 153–165.

43. E. T. Lee, et al., "A follow-up study of diabetic Oklahoma Indians," *Diabetes Care*, Supplement (1993): 300–305.

44. W. T. Boyce, et al., "Sociocultural factors in puerperal infectious morbidity among Navajo women," *Am. J. Epidemiol.* 129 (1989): 604–615.

45. T. A. Cullen, et al., "Chlamydia trachomatic infection in Native American women in a southwestern tribe," *J. Fam. Practice* 31 (1990): 552–554.

46. T. M. Becker, et al., "Cervical papillomavirus infection and cervical dysplasia in Hispanic, Native American, and Non-Hispanic White women in New Mexico," *Am. J. Public Health* 81 (1991): 582–586.

47. R. L. Hall, et al., "Assessment of AIDS knowledge, attitudes, behaviors, and risk level of Northwestern American Indians," *Am. J. Public Health* 80 (1990): 875–877.

48. J. Sugarman, et al., "Tuberculosis among American Indians and Alaska Natives, 1985–1990," *The Provider* 16 (1991): 186–190.

49. G. A. Conway, et al., "Prevalence of HIV and AIDS in American Indians and Alaskan Natives," *The Provider* 17 (1992): 65–70.

50. P. A. May, K. J. Hymbaugh, and J. M. Aase, "Epidemiology of fetal alcohol syndrome among American Indians of the Southwest," *Soc. Biol.* 30 (1983): 374–387.

51. K. B. Masis and P. A. May, "A comprehensive local program for the prevention of fetal alcohol syndrome," *Public Health Report* 106 (1991): 484–489.

52. R. H. Jarrell, "Native American women and forced sterilization, 1973–1976," *Caduceus*, Winter (1992): 45–58.

53. B. C. Milligan, "Patient's rights and sterilizations," *The Provider* 18 (1993): 36–37.

54. M. D. Brown, "Norplant: The newest reversible contraceptive," *The Provider* 18 (1993): 17–19.

55. W. L. Dienst, "Subdermal contraceptive implants in the IHS: The Crow service unit experience," *The Provider* 18 (1992): 20–31.

56. G. Brenneman, C. Vanderwagen, and J. Porvaznik, "Infant mortality among American Indian and Alaska Native populations: Successes and challenges," *Children Today* 19 (1990): 21–25.

57. R. M. Nakamura, et al., "Excess infant mortality in an American Indian population, 1940–1990," *JAMA* 266 (1991): 2244–2248.

58. W. T. Boyce, et al., "Social and cultural factors in pregnancy complications among Navajo women," *Am. J. Epidemiol.* 124 (1986): 242–253.

59. S. C. Lapham, E. Henley, and K. Kleyboecker, "Prenatal behavioral risk screening by computer among Native Americans," *Fam. Med.* 25 (1993): 197–202.

60. B. C. Campbell, et al., "Using 1990 National MCH objectives to assess health status and risk in an American Indian community," *Public Health Report* 104 (1989): 627–631.

61. A. M. Michalek and M. C. Mahoney, "Cancer in native populations: Lessons to be learned," *J. Cancer Educ.* 5 (1990): 243–249.

62. M. C. Mahoney and A. M. Michalek, "A meta-analysis of cancer incidence in United States and Canadian native populations," *Int. J. Epidemiol.* 20 (1991): 323–327.

63. E. R. Rhoades, "The major respiratory diseases of American Indians," *Am. Rev. Resp. Dis.* 141 (1990): 595–600.

64. E. T. Lee, et al., "The Strong Heart Study. A study of cardiovascular disease in American Indians: Design and methods," *Am. J. Epidemiol.* 132 (1990): 1141–1155.

65. B. V. Howard, et al., "Risk factors for coronary heart disease in diabetic and nondiabetic Native Americans," *Diabetes* 41 (1992): 4–11.

66. S. H. Nelson, et al., "An overview of mental health services for American Indians and Alaska Natives in the 1990s," *Hospital and Community Psychiatry* 43 (1992): 257–261.

67. N. W. Van Winkle and P. A. May, "An update on American Indian suicide in New Mexico, 1980–87," *Hum. Org.* 52 (1993): 304–315.

68. R. D. Walker, et al., "Treatment implications of comorbid psychopathology in American Indians and Alaska Natives," *Culture, Medicine and Psychiatry* 16 (1993): 555–572.

69. J. L. Shore, et al., "A pilot study of depression among American Indian patients with Research Diagnostic Criteria," *Am. Ind. Alaska Native Ment. Health Res.* 1 (1987): 4–15.

70. J. D. Kinzie, et al., "Psychiatric epidemiology of an Indian village: A nineteen-year study," *J. Nerv. Ment. Dis.* 180 (1992): 33–39.

71. R. D. Walker, personal communication, Aug. 30, 1993.

72. T. Burns, "Data abstract—Alcoholism Treatment Guidance System," Aug. 30, 1993.

73. P. A. May, "Substance abuse and American Indians: An overview," *Int. J. Addict.* 17 (1982): 1185–1209.

74. S. Z. Kunitz, *Disease Change and the Role of Medicine: The Navajo Experience.* 1983, Berkeley, CA: University of California Press.

75. J. C. Weibel-Orlando, J. Long, and T. S. Weisner, *A Comparison of Urban and Rural Indian Drinking Patterns in California.* 1982, Los Angeles: Alcohol Research Center, UCLA Neuropsychiatric Institute.

76. Indian Health Service, *Trends in Indian Health, 1990.* 1990, Rockville, MD: U.S. Department of Health and Human Services.

77. L. J. D. Wallace and R. J. Smith, "Injury prevention in the Indian Health Service: A role for primary care providers," *The Provider* 17 (1992): 193–198.

78. A Hill, "Treatment and prevention of alcoholism in the Native American family," in *Alcoholism and Substance Abuse in Special Populations,* G. W. Lawson and A. W. Lawson, editors. 1989, Rockville, MD: Aspen Publishers, Inc. Pp. 247–272.

79. T. C. Harford, "Family history of alcoholism in the United States: Prevalence and demographic characteristics," *Brit. J. Addict.* 87 (1992): 931–935.

80. R. G. Thwaites, *Jesuit Relations and Allied Documents 1601–1791.* 1896–1901, Cleveland: Burrows Brothers.

81. D. Fenna, et al., "Ethanol metabolism in various racial groups," *Can. Med. Assoc. J.* 105 (1971): 472–475.

82. J. A. Ewing, B. A. Rouse, and E. D. Pellizzari, "Alcohol sensitivity and ethnic background," *Am. J. Psychiatry* 131 (1974): 206–210.

83. L. J. Bennion and T. K. Li, "Alcohol metabolism in American Indians and whites: Lack of racial differences in metabolic rate and liver alcohol dehydrogenase," *New Engl. J. Med.* 294 (1976): 9–13.

84. J. M. Hanna, "Ethnic groups, human variation, and alcohol use," in *Cross-Cultural Approaches to Study of Alcohol,* M. W. Everett, J. O. Waddell, and D. B. Heath, editors. 1976, Mouton: The Hague. Pp. 235–242.

85. J. J. Farris and B. M. Jones, "Ethanol metabolism in male American Indians and whites," *Alcoholism: Clin. Exp. Res.* 2 (1977): 77–81.

86. C. S. Lieber, "Metabolism of ethanol and alcoholism: Racial and acquired factors," *Ann. Intern. Med.* 76 (1972): 326–327.

87. P. H. Wolff, "Ethnic differences in alcohol sensitivity," *Science* 175 (1972): 449–450.

88. T. E. Reed, et al., "Alcohol acetaldehyde metabolism in Caucasian, Chinese, and Amerinds," *Can. Med. Assoc. J.* 115 (1976): 851–855.

89. A. R. Zeiner, A. Paredes, and L. Cowden, "Physiological responses to ethanol among the Tarahumara Indians," *Ann. N. Y. Acad. Sci.* 273 (1976): 151–158.

90. A. R. Zeiner, A. Paredes, and H. D. Christiansen, "The role of acetaldehyde in mediating reactivity to an acute dose of ethanol among different racial groups," *Alcohol: Clin. Exp. Res.* 2 (1979): 11–18.

91. N. K. Mello, "Etiological theories of alcoholism" in *Advances in Substance Abuse,* N. K. Mello, editor. 1983, Greenwich, CT: JAI Press. Pp. 271–312.

92. J. M. Schaefer, "Ethnic and racial variations in alcohol use and abuse," in *Special Population Issues.* DHHS Publication No. (ADM) 82-1193, NIAAA, editor. 1982, Washington, DC: U.S. Government Printing Office. Pp. 293–311.

93. J. Leland, *Firewater Myths: North american Indian Drinking and Alcohol Addiction.* 1976, New Brunswick, NJ: Rutgers Center of Alcohol Studies.

94. J. Leland, "Native American alcohol use: A review of the literature," in *From Tulapai to Tokay: A Bibliography of Alcohol Use and Abuse among Native Americans of North America,* P. D. Mail and D. R. McDonald, editors. 1980, New Haven, CT: HRAF Press. Pp. 1–56.

95. D. Goldman, et al., "DRD2 dopamine receptor genotype, linkage disequilibrium, and alcoholism in American Indians and other populations," *Alcohol Clin. Exp. Res.* 17 (1993): 199–204.

96. T. L. Wall, et al., "Alcohol and aldehyde dehydrogenase genotypes and family history of alcoholism," in *Proceedings of the Research Society on Alcoholism Annual Meeting.* 1993. San Antonio, TX.

97. C. Garcia-Andrade, et al., "Response to alcohol in Native American men with and without a family history of alcoholism," in *Proceedings of the Research Society on Alcoholism Annual Meeting.* 1993. San Antonio, TX.

98. C. L. Ehlers, et al., "EEG fast frequency activity and alcoholism risk in Native American men," in *Proceedings of the Research Society on Alcoholism Annual Meeting.* 1993. San Antonio, TX.

99. D. H. Van Thiel and J. S. Gavaler, "Ethanol metabolism and hepatotoxicity: Does sex make a difference?" in *Recent Developments in Alcoholism,* M. Galanter, editor. 1988, New York: Plenum Press. Pp. 291–304.

100. M. Frezza, C. Di Padova, and G. Pozzato, "The role of decreased gastric alcohol dehydrogenase activity and first-pass metabolism," *N. Engl. J. Med.* 322 (1990): 95–99.

101. W. El-Sadr and L. Capps, "The challenge of minority recruitment in clinical trials for AIDS," *JAMA* 267 (1992): 954–957.

102. D. Britten and J. R. Sugarman, "Year 2000 objectives for STDs: the IHS Portland area approach," *The Provider* 18 (1993): 91–94.

103. G. A. Conway, "Racial misclassification of AI/AN patients with class IV HIV infection," *The Provider* 17 (1992): 72.

Ethical and Legal Issues Relating to the Inclusion of Asian/Pacific Islanders in Clinical Studies

Elena S. H. Yu

A precise count of Asian and Pacific Islander Americans (APIAs) is lacking. According to the 1990 Census, the official count of APIAs is only 7.3 million. However, according to the *Healthy People 2000* report (U.S. Department of Human Services, 1990), there are more than 11 million APIAs. Regardless of what the number is, the consensus exists that APIAs are the fastest growing ethnic minority in America, followed by Hispanics. Between 1980 and 1990, they increased by 108%, with California surpassing the national rate and growing by 127%. Indeed, every state except Hawaii sustained a growth rate of at least 40%. The slower rate of increase in Hawaii (17%) is attributable to the fact that the Asian/Pacific Islanders represent three-fifths of the population in that state. Already, immigrants from Asia on average form about 45% of all immigrants entering the United States annually. Despite this phenomenal increase, APIAs remain the most underresearched and the least understood ethnic minority in America.

The purpose of this paper is to complement some of the points made in the paper by Gamble (1994) and to present an Asian/Pacific Islander *minority* perspective to the ethical and legal issues of including APIA populations in clinical studies. A description of the APIA population is presented below, followed by a general overview of the sources of epidemiologic and health data on this special ethnic minority. Next, several conceptual and methodological issues are identified and discussed. They include: (1) problems in the definition of the study population; (2) the myth of a healthy minority; (3) lack of baseline epidemiologic data on ethnic subgroups; (4) dissemination of information from existing studies; and (5) the issue of informed consent. Implicit in these discussions is the need to empower APIA minority investigators in research, in order to foster cultural sensitivity in research and to ensure that the objectives of clinical studies will benefit both minority and majority populations alike.

DESCRIPTION OF THE POPULATION

The term Asian/Pacific Islander Americans encompasses at least 45 ethnic groups. Nationally, Asian Americans make up about 95% of the APIA population and Pacific Islanders about 5%. Among Asians, Chinese and Filipinos—with about 1.6 and 1.4 million members, respectively—are the two largest subpopulations, comprising 23% and 19% respectively of the total APIA population. They are followed by the Japanese (12%), Asian Indians (11%), and Koreans (11%), each numbering near or over 800,000. Vietnamese form the smallest percentage (8%) of the six major APIA subgroups. Insofar as the Pacific Islander populations are concerned, Hawaiians are the largest group, with over 200,000 persons, followed by the Samoans and Guamanians (63,000 and 49,000, respectively), and then by Tongans and Fijians, who number less than 20,000 and 10,000, respectively.

Unique Characteristics of the APIA Population

In 1990, a majority of the APIAs resided in just three states: California, New York, and Hawaii. Seventy-nine percent of all APIAs may be found in 10 states (California, New York, Hawaii, Texas, Illinois, New Jersey, Washington, Virginia, Florida, and Massachusetts). More detailed information from the 1990 Census by ethnicity for the APIAs is not yet available. What little aggregate demographic data that exist point to the following conclusions. Within this special population, some ethnic groups, such as Japanese Americans, are reported to have annual family incomes 38 percent higher than the national median income (APPCHO, 1993). Other groups, such as Laotian immigrants, have one of the highest poverty rates of any group in the nation (U.S. Department of Human Services, 1990). These family income data obscure the fact that Asian Americans and Pacific Islanders have larger numbers of family members living together than the general U.S. population and that it is a cultural practice to pool the income of household members in order to cover family expenses.

There are several other unique characteristics about this special population. First, they are geographically concentrated and yet widely dispersed. Some 58.5% live in the Western regions of the United States, 17.4% live in the Northeast, 13.8% live in the South, and 10.3% live in the Midwest. About 45% of the APIA population live inside central cities, compared with 25% of the white American population. Only 6% of the APIAs live in nonmetropolitan areas, compared with 24% for white Americans. However, within the continental United States, APIAs represent less than 10% of the total state population of California and even smaller percentages in the remaining 9 states with the largest APIA population. This special population is also predominantly foreign-born rather than U.S.-born. As a result, a significantly large percentage of the population do not speak English fluently. Many are linguistically isolated—defined as the absence of any household member, 14 years and older, who can speak English.

SOURCES OF EPIDEMIOLOGIC AND HEALTH DATA

Health and epidemiologic data on APIAs are severely limited for a number of reasons, such as: (1) many research data, including those collected by the federal government, on APIAs cannot be further stratified by ethnic groups; (2) where the data have been coded to identify specific ethnic groups, as in the U.S. vital statistics records, the number of groups that can be identified are limited only to the older immigrants or Pacific Islander populations [changes are now being introduced by the National Center for Health Statistics (NCHS) to expand the codes for the APIA subgroups]; (3) local or regional studies of Asian Americans and Pacific Islanders are very few and seldom published in widely accessible journals. These studies limit generalizability because of the profound diversity within APIA populations. Consequently, we know little about the health problems of APIAs other than those that have been commonly reported for some time. We know from *Healthy People 2000* that:

> the breast cancer incidence rate among Native Hawaiians is 111 per 100,000 women, as compared to 86 per 100,000 among whites. The lung cancer rate is 18 percent higher among Southeast Asian men than for the white population. And the liver cancer rate is more than 12 times higher among Southeast Asians than in the white population. Higher rates of high blood pressure have been found among Filipinos aged 50 and older living in California than among the total California population.

We also know from the California data that the leading causes of death for Asians and Pacific Islanders are: heart disease (28%), cancer (24%), stroke (9%), injuries (79%), pneumonia/influenza (4%), chronic lung disease (3%), suicide (2%), diabetes (2%), perinatal conditions (2%), and liver disease (1%). Tuberculosis and hepatitis B are the two major infectious diseases that afflict large segments of the APIA population. Smoking is the single most significant "lifestyle" factor that poses a threat to their health. Among the California immigrant groups, smoking rates among men are 92% for Laotians, 71% for Cambodians, and 65% for Vietnamese compared to 30% for the overall

American population. Moreover, since an overwhelming majority of the immigrant groups are foreign-born, linguistic and cultural issues are persistent barriers to health care as well.

The increasing economic power of the Pacific Rim countries and the shift in U.S. funding policies towards supporting more studies on under-studied populations, such as women and minorities, mean that Asian Americans and Pacific Islanders have finally become the new frontiers of research explorations when they have been a historically ignored subject pool in past studies. The interest in Asian Americans and Pacific Islanders as a potential source of study subjects comes at a time when medical and public health professions are advocating for more clinical trials. The benefits to mankind and to the scientific community of being able to do research in experimentally controlled settings are obvious. Unfortunately, a number of factors—such as the historical backgrounds of Asian/Pacific Islanders' immigration to the United States, the sociocultural contexts of their medical manpower development, and the past history of medical research in Asia and the Pacific Islands, significantly affects how individuals in this special population will *perceive and interpret* the new research emphasis. Lack of knowledge about how to define and identify the different subpopulations of APIAs, ignorance of the morbidity risks of this ethnic minority, and lack of baseline epidemiologic data also severely constrain the scientific justification for clinical studies, especially clinical trials.

Historical Factors and Manpower Development

From 1882, when the Anti-Chinese Exclusion Act was passed to prevent Chinese from entering the United States and becoming citizens, to the Gentlemen's Agreement of 1906 that curbed Japanese immigration, and the 1924 Immigration Act prohibiting the entry of "aliens ineligible for citizenship"—which included the entire Asia-Pacific basin all the way to Greece—up until 1965, Asian/Pacific Islanders have been systematically treated as *less desirable* than white Europeans. Today, despite the impressive academic achievements of Asian Americans in SAT-quantitative tests at the high school level (they perform poorly on the SAT-English tests, which is seldom noted by the media), and despite alleged "overrepresentation" of Asian Americans in medical schools, few Asian Americans and even fewer Pacific Islanders have made it into *medical research fields*. The small numbers cannot possibly be merely a random process when one takes into consideration the size of the denominator or population of Asian Americans who completed medical training or have a Ph.D. degree in public health, compared to other ethnic groups. We know from diverse sources that between 1973 and 1992, the representation of APIAs among all applicants to medical schools increased from 1.3 percent to

16.5 percent (Association of American Medical Colleges, 1993). Among those who applied to medical schools, acceptance rates for Asian Americans have ranged from a low of 28 percent during the 1974–75 academic year to a high of 63.4 percent during the 1988–89 academic year, and now are 50.6 percent for the 1991–92 academic year. Between 1977 and 1992, the number of APIAs enrolled in medical schools increased from 1,422 to 9,438, or from 2.4% to 14.4%. In terms of medical school graduates, the number is smaller. Available data showed that only 378 APIAs graduated from medical schools in the 1978–79 academic year, and by 1990–91 that number increased to 1,687. Still, the percentage of APIAs who graduated from U.S. medical schools has increased significantly during these two periods, from 2.6% of total graduates in 1978–79 to 10.9 percent of total graduates in 1990–91 (Gall and Gall, 1993). These figures do not include graduates of schools of public health, for which data are not available. Notwithstanding the large numbers of Asian Americans who completed M.D., D.Sc., or Ph.D. degrees, few made their careers in academia or in research as principal investigators (PIs) of large projects. They often appear as research associates or as technical experts, rarely as co-PIs, thereby having very little impact on broad health policy decisions. Thus, the medical *research* profession itself, being historically dominated by mainstream white-American investigators, now has a new mission—to increase the participation of women and minorities as *subjects* in clinical trials. Does any Asian/Pacific Islander have any problem with that?

Factors Affecting Data Interpretation in Clinical Trials

In the process of designing and conducting clinical trials, a number of factors which affect the interpretation of data need to be fully articulated. This author considers the following issues important.

Definition of the Study Population

The term Asian Americans and Pacific Islanders covers a myriad of cultures and at least 45 linguistic groups whose ancestries can be traced to places that include Mongolia to the north, the islands near Australia to the south, India and Pakistan to the west, and Hawaii to the east. In terms of skin color, this population consists of a full-range of "colors," ranging from "black" to "brown," "yellow," and "white." For example, the Spaniards who have settled in the Philippines and who considered themselves Filipinos are "white" by skin pigmentation, while the *Spanish mestizas* who are of mixed parentage may be of any mix of colors. No existing racial classification schemes can possibly identify the members of this population into only one racial stock or gene pool. In their native habitats, some are nomads living on horseback; others ride the "bullet trains" that even the United States does not have; and still others go to work in chauffer-driven Rolls Royces. In terms of indigenous diet, some are vegetarians, others shun pork, while still others do not eat beef. Suffice it to say that they differ immensely in terms of racial origin, religion, lifestyle, diet, and health. How does one scientifically define this special population in any piece of epidemiologic and clinical research? What should one use as the criteria for determining whether someone is an Asian/Pacific Islander or a member of a subgroup of its populations, such as Chinese, Japanese, Filipinos, Hawaiians, Samoans, Guamanians or others? Should the definition be based on ancestry? Self-definition of ethnicity? Or interviewer observation of "race," as has occurred in several government surveys prior to 1976? And how should one "treat" or interpret findings of "racial" differences between white and APIA populations? Unless these basic conceptual issues are handled carefully, any clinical study which reports data for APIAs without additional breakdowns by ethnicity is subject to distortions and misinterpretations. Definitions based on "race" may be useful in research on genetics and disease (if a consensus can be reached on the validity and reliability of any existing "racial classification" systems), but the same classification system may not be useful if the critical determinant of health or disease is in fact lifestyle and not genes. In the latter case, being able to classify the study subjects in terms of their *ethnic group identity* may be preferred to "race," for the former would shed light on the group membership and normative lifestyles of the study subjects that may be salient in explaining a particular health outcome.

The Myth of a Healthy Minority

Due to lack of research and inadequate information, findings from available studies on APIAs may have unwittingly sustained the *myth*—begun in the 1960s—that Asian Americans are quite healthy compared with black or white Americans. The best known investigator-initiated studies of Asian Americans conducted in Hawaii and California are "migrant studies"—which are by nature comparative. Typically, a specific population—usually the Japanese—are sampled in three locations (e.g., Japan, Hawaii, and California) and compared, or they are studied in two locations (e.g., Japan and Hawaii, or Japan and California) and then compared to white Americans. Using similar study designs and questionnaires to the extent possible, inferences are drawn about the health status or morbidity patterns of the Japanese as an example of Asian/Pacific Islanders. While logically sound, an unintended consequence of this approach is to use the most established Asian American subgroup—which happens to have an extremely large percentage of English speakers and also the highest socioeconomic attainment of all Asian Americans—to represent *the* APIAs—an ethnic minority characterized by a heavy representation of persons from low socioeconomic status and nonnative English speakers. Thus, it is easy for both the media and policymakers to gloss over the issue of ethnic diversity in health and morbidity. Furthermore, comparisons between the Japanese and white Americans have often led to the conclusion that the Japanese are in "better" health than white Americans. They may have inadvertently buoyed the *myth* of Asians as a healthy minority, at the expense of rigorously controlling for social class or socioeconomic status—a key variable in any health study. In several epidemiologic studies of Asian subgroups, social class or socioeconomic status have often been poorly measured, even if they can be and have been properly "controlled for" statistically. Consequently, the general public or mainstream researchers are not always aware that the other APIA subgroups are very much *unlike* the Japanese Americans. Often, use of the term APIA confers a myth of cultural and racial homogeneity, which in turn gives the appearance of scientific validity when in fact the numbers of specific APIA subgroups included in past population-based studies conducted in the United States have been extremely small to the point of being insignificant and unanalyzable.

Yu and Liu (1992) have noted that our knowledge of the health risks and morbidity patterns of different Asian/Pacific Islander subgroups in the United States have been drawn primarily from the following general sources of data: (1) investigator-initiated epidemiologic surveys conducted in Hawaii and at the West Coast, such as the migrant studies described above and other types of studies (Curb et al., 1991; Kagan et al., 1974; Kato, Tillotson, Nichaman, Rhaods, and Robertson et al., 1977; Stavig, Igra, and Leonard, 1984; Stemmermann, Chyou, Kagan, Nomura, and Yano, 1991; Takeya et al., 1984; Tillotson et al., 1973; Yano and MacLean, 1989; Yano, Reed, Curb, Hankin, and Albers, 1986); (2) Surveillance, Epidemiology and End Results (SEER) cancer registry data maintained in selected cities (Hinds, Kolonel, Lee, and Hirohata, 1980; Kolonel et al., 1981; Yu, 1986); (3) descriptive clinic-based studies, such as the Kaiser Permanente Prepaid Health Plan (Angel, Armstrong, and Klatsky, 1989; Klatsky and Armstrong, 1991); and (4) mortality statistics compiled by the National Center for Health Statistics (Haenszel and Kurihara, 1968; King, 1975; Kleinman, 1990; Li, Ni, Schwartz, and Daling, 1990; Liu and Yu, 1985; Lynberg and Muin, 1990; Yu, 1982). There have been extremely few *clinical studies*, much less *clinical trials* involving APIAs. Of the few that exist, most are focused primarily on pharmacologic reactions. Usually, only one subpopulation is studied, although the word "Asian" may be used in the reports, thereby giving the false impression of validity and generalizability to the entire APIA population. This quantum jump in logical inference from one subgroup to "all" Asian/Pacific Islanders should be avoided. Instead, the subpopulation should be specifically identified.

Lack of Baseline Epidemiologic Data on Ethnic Subgroups

In the absence of alternative data sources, continuing use of the existing data and implicit acceptance of their methodological approaches have had at least two negative consequences: (1) a slower rate of development of knowledge about the morbidity risks more commonly encountered in Asian/Pacific Islander subgroups than in the majority white population; and (2) a general lack of baseline data on Asian/Pacific Islander ethnic groups and health status.

As scientists continue to use the prevailing morbidity risks of white or black Americans as the basis for research, scientific and public awareness of more troubling Asian American health risks (e.g., tuberculosis and hepatitis B, stroke and diabetes) remained low until the media recognized that these diseases are affecting the mainstream populations at an alarming rate. What are the common diseases that Asian/Pacific Islanders experience besides the ones listed above? Will the informed APIA investigators succeed in drawing attention to the importance of studying diseases that might be more prevalent and have a higher incidence in their ethnic communities than in the mainstream society? And will their effort to study ethnic-specific diseases be encouraged through grant awards or will we continue to study diseases that are epidemiologically far more common in, or which have a greater impact on, the mainstream population than in the APIA communities?

The most fundamental problem with the new push to include APIA population in clinical trials is the near total absence of a descriptive database about these vulnerable populations that could provide a scientific basis for their inclusion. Clinical studies, and specially clinical trials, by design involve far more risk than *mere* descriptive surveys. The potential for ethnic misunderstandings is great because the scientific community, which is predominantly white, and which previously showed lack of interest in collecting descriptive epidemiologic data on the APIA populations, now encourages the inclusion of minorities in their clinical trials. Progress in research has no doubt been made, but nagging questions will continue to haunt us. Questions such as: Why is it not important to collect baseline data on these underresearched populations? Who would benefit most from clinical studies—the majority population or the minorities? Which diseases or health conditions are targeted for clinical trials? Are there diseases that afflict the APIA populations in strikingly larger proportions than the mainstream U.S. populations (e.g., cancer, stroke, atherosclerosis, thinness in some subpopulations and obesity in other groups, normal cholesterol levels but abnormal triglycerides)? Or are there health conditions which impact more severely on the mainstream white populations than on the APIA minorities, in terms of proportional mortality? Who decides what specific diseases should be studied in clinical trials? Who benefits the most from these clinical studies? What is the ethnic composition of the peer review committees who approve the grant applications for clinical trials? To what extent have ethical criteria been incorporated into the peer review process?

The invasiveness of clinical trials, compared to what are known as "observational studies" in epidemiology or population-based door-to-door survey types of research in the social sciences, raises the spectre of *mass* experimentation and highlights the *dispensability* of the APIA population. The existing poverty in many subgroups of APIAs will make them exceedingly vulnerable to the temptations of submitting themselves as human subjects for clinical trials in exchange for monetary rewards. Often, offers of $200 to $800 payments, fairly common in clinical trials that involve the collection of biological specimens, far exceed the one-month take-home pay of individuals living in poverty. Because of this, the issue of informed consent in vulnerable populations must be deliberated, and the legal liability and moral responsibility issues must be studied carefully. Should legal liabilities not extend a lifetime when the effects of some drugs, such as steroids and hormones, might be life long? How do we determine what is the appropriate length of follow-up for clinical trials? How do we clarify the moral responsibility of researchers to keep their subjects informed of their research findings? Who owns the clinical data collected by the investigators? Moreover, how do we ensure and enforce informed consent in clinical trials?

Dissemination of Information from Existing Studies

A few studies have been conducted on Asians and Pacific Islanders in their home countries as part of the U.S. involvement in the Pacific theatre or as a consequence of its foreign policies. But findings from such studies are not widely known, even though they have been reported in peer-reviewed journals.

For example, some of the U.S. military's activities and observations of Pacific Islanders are widely known to the public only through coverage by the media. CBS, for instance, once broadcast (on 60 Minutes, CBS Television Network, July 13, 1980) that the U.S. government had conducted 43 separate nuclear explosions mainly on the Pacific atoll of Eniwetok, which consists of 41 named islands and is part of the now independent Marshall Islands. These nuclear events resulted in serious contamination with plutonium, strontium, cesium, and other dangerous substances on the northern islands of Eniwetok where the bombs were exploded. The inhabitants were relocated to another island. Six inches of contaminated topsoil and tons of radioactive metal from test towers were removed bargeload by bargeload, to be buried in one island called Runit, making the latter off limits for the next 24,000 years. The clean-up has theoretically removed the plutonium; but beneath the plutonium-free soil, "there is still cesium and strontium and one or two other elements that are hazardous to your health" (CBS News, 1980:14). The Eniwetok explosion is similar to an earlier U.S. bombing experience on Bikini Island, which has provided ample evidence that local vegetations, such as coconuts, continue to contain high levels of cesium and strontium, despite any nuclear clean-up efforts. The inhabitants who returned to live on Bikini Island showed high traces of plutonium in their bodies and run a high risk of getting cancer. Hence, they had to be removed once again from the island and are "forever wards of the United States" (CBS News, 1980). But, when the people of Eniwetoks demanded to return to their native land, the U.S. military facilitated their return. A dose assessment team was assembled by the United States, presumably to inform the inhabitants "who've never seen an electric light bulb" about the risks of living on the contaminated atolls. It was clear from the 60 Minutes report that the U.S. military kept good records of the Bikini Island inhabitants and intended to do the same with the Eniwetok islanders. But has the scientific community been able to evaluate these data? And did the inhabitants of the affected atolls really know what had taken place in their lives? Can a population with about a fourth-grade level of education and one that lives in a subsistence economy have informed knowledge about the devastating long-term impact of radiation on human physiology and functioning? Is this or is this not "natural" experimentation with human subjects conducted under the guise of "humanitarian" clean-up efforts and medical "follow ups"?

The above questions attain a certain degree of significance when one considers that the first human subjects to be used in the testing of the effectiveness of the pill as a method of contraception were poor women in Puerto Rico during the early 1960s. Poverty was the social and ethical justification for selecting Puerto Rican women into the early trials on the effectiveness of the pill as a contraceptive device. By the late 1970s, we would learn from scientific studies conducted in the People's Republic of China that the dosage of specific hormones in the pill produced in the United States were "unnecessarily high." Now, of course, we also know the potential adverse impact of these hormones on the development of certain types of diseases (e.g., thromboembolism). But where are the poor Puerto Rican women now who were the human subjects for the clinical studies of the "pill" 20–30 years ago? Given the current knowledge that the latency period for some diseases may be more than 10 years—some may be 20 years or longer—did the clinical trials on the pill in the 1960s play an important role in the reportedly high incidence of many diseases among Puerto Rican women today? There was a legal reason for choosing Puerto Rico as the site for U.S. clinical studies (it was part of the United States and yet some U.S. laws on drug testings did not apply to the island). What is the legal liability of the investigators to the Puerto Rican subjects 20 years or more after the clinical trials have been completed? Few pharmaceutical companies run their clinical trials over a long period of time. Rather, the trials are cut off as soon as a particular "positive" or "beneficial" effect has been "substantiated" by an acceptable p-value. This deliberate cut-off of the length of observation in clinical studies, prompted no doubt by the twin forces of funding constraints and pressure to market a new drug, means that the *long-term effects* of many drugs tested in clinical trials remain unknown. The moral responsibility to make a drug available to the public as soon as it is found to be effective in the treatment of a disease must be balanced by the moral obligation to establish built-in follow-up procedures over a long-term period in order to determine unanticipated side effects or to monitor the subjects' health on a continuing basis. Now, does the absence of knowledge about the long-term effects of a drug or surgical procedure justify the absence of medical and legal measures to follow up the subjects for life? As Puerto Ricans become more aware of their rights, will other territories under U.S. possession located in the Pacific Ocean become even more convenient sites for many risky clinical trials involving human subjects? In the context of these concerns, the Institute of Medicine's effort to understand the legal and ethical issues of including Asian and Pacific Islanders in clinical trials is commendable. In what follows, we discuss the problems of obtaining informed consent from Asian Americans and Pacific Islanders, leaving aside the issue of legal liabilities because of lack of expertise on this subject.

The Issue of Informed Consent

The concept of informed consent, adopted by the USPHS in medical experiments only in 1966, refers to a person's ability to consent freely to participate in a study in which he or she adequately understands both what is required and the "cost" or risk for participating in the study (Wolfensberger, 1967). On July 12, 1974, the National Research Act (Pub. L. 93-348) was signed into law, thereby creating the National Commission on the Protection of Human Subjects of Biomedical and Behavioral Research. The latter produced the Belmont Report (U.S. Department of Human Services, 1979), which identifies the basic ethical principles for research with human subjects and established guidelines which should be followed to assure that such research is conducted in accordance with those principles. The Public Health Service Act, as amended by the Health Research Extension Act of 1985 Public Law 99-158 (November 20, 1985) specifies the details for the establishment of Institutional Review Boards at institutions where research on human subjects are to be conducted. The Code of Federal Regulations, Title 45, Part 46 (U.S. Department of Human Services, revised June 18, 1991), further spells out the meaning of informed consent, the types of research requiring informed consent, and the kind of information that is required to establish informed consent. These successive instances of legislation provide evidence of formal and legal protection of human subjects in research. However, how these laws are implemented in the informal context of everyday life is far from clear.

Yu and Liu (1986) pointed out that under normal conditions and with Americans who have had more than 40 years of exposure to polls, surveys, and clinical trials, the task of obtaining informed consent is a routine procedure. But in dealing with special populations such as the poor, the uneducated, and recent immigrants and refugees from Asia and the Pacific Islands, chances are great that for one reason or another, a sizable number are unable to absorb the information necessary for them to meaningfully grant informed consent, even where the interviewers are "racially" matched with the study subjects (Hurh and Kim, 1982). The problem of informed consent is more serious among the APIA population than among black Americans in the sense that many Asians and Pacific Islanders, being predominantly foreign-born, lack a general idea of what their basic human rights are in this country. For a large majority, freedom of political expression never existed in their country of origin. Some segments of the population, particularly older women, are least able to express themselves, assert their rights, or ask questions (Yu and Liu, 1986: 487). Not having been included often enough as subjects in the major descriptive epidemiologic studies in the United States, APIAs are naturally unfamiliar with the expectations and procedures, promises, and limitations of medical and public health research. Several investigators have noted, though not published, their observations that some APIA study subjects will sign their name because the *source* that asked them to do so is credible and *not* because they understand what was asked of them or the risks involved. A credible source includes such individuals as professors or doctors, who, in traditional APIA cultures are revered and cannot be questioned. To date, there has not been any systematic study of how APIAs understand the process of informed consent in research in general, or in specific types of studies such as survey interviews versus clinical trials. The high illiteracy rate among older APIA women means that even when the informed consent form is written in their native non-English language, a significantly large number of them will still not be able to understand the words they see nor can they sign their name. Will majority and minority investigators be trained in the ethics of obtaining informed consent from such "vulnerable" populations? How will the regulations for ensuring informed consent be enforced?

DISCUSSION

In a nutshell, a lack of baseline epidemiologic studies on APIAs based on representative samples leaves us without adequate knowledge of the diversity in culture and health of this special population. The low cholesterol levels of the Japanese serve as useful references for the control of coronary heart disease in mainstream America, but has the lesson been learned and disseminated as widely with regards to the high risk of stroke among the Japanese? And have we focused sufficient attention on the control of trigylcerides among APIAs in order to reduce, possibly, their risk for strokes—a disease which strikes APIAs at a higher proportion than white Americans? These questions illustrate the importance of collecting baseline epidemiologic data on specific ethnic populations and the value of understanding why a piece of epidemiologic research is undertaken, who it benefits, and what uses are made of the findings. These are clearly politically charged issues, ones that would become even more so if left unattended.

A striking contrast between the black American's and the APIA's perspectives on the legal and ethical issues in clinical studies is that while black - Americans have had a history of slavery and have been the object of abuses in medical research (the Tuskegee Syphilis Study being the most glaring of such violations), APIAs suffer from just the opposite—a lack of studies based on representative samples that would adequately reflect the cultural diversity of this special population and inform us of their most troubling health conditions. Consequently, the few studies that exist, which were based on the most economically successful group—the Japanese—and the most accessible one—because they primarily speak English—are used to overgeneralize "all" APIAs. Social class differences between the Japanese and white American populations are seldom rigorously controlled such that observed differences are quickly attributed to basic "racial" differences when in fact they may be socioeconomic in nature.

In the absence of any good descriptive baseline data about Asian Americans and Pacific Islanders, and evidence of an inadequate record of training minorities to become principal investigators of large-scale studies, the USPHS effort to include a large sample of APIA populations in clinical studies is scientifically premature and viewed with considerable suspicion by the educated members of the APIA community. Every effort must be made to answer the fundamental question—*research for what purpose and to whose benefit?*—before embarking on any major clinical trials involving vulnerable populations. More minority investigators will have to be trained and become equal partners of research with mainstream investigators in order to ensure the representation of minority perspectives in research.

REFERENCES

AAPCHO (Association of Asian Pacific Community Health Organizations): 1993. *Community Health Watch* 1(2).

Angel, A., Armstrong, M.A., and Klatsky, A.L. 1989. Blood pressure among Asian-Americans living in Northern Califonia. *American Journal of Cardiology* 64:237–240.

Association of American Medical Colleges. 1993 AAMC Data Book: Statistical Information Related to Medical Education. Washington, D.C.: Association of American Medical Colleges.

Bureau of the Census. 1991. Race and Hispanic Origin. 1990 Census Profile Number 2, June 1991. Washington, D.C.: U.S. Department of Commerce.

CBS News: Remember Eniwetok? 60 Minutes, Vol. XII, Number 44, as broadcast over CBS Television Network, Sunday, July 13, 1980, 7:00–8:00 p.m., EDT, with CBS News Correspondents Mike Wallace, Morley Safer, Dan Rather, and Harry Reasoner, pp. 1–17. Copyright MCMLXXX CBS Inc.

Curb, J.D., Aluli, N.E., Kautz, J.A., Petrovitch, H., Knutsen, S.F., Knutsen, R., O'Conner, H.K., and O'Conner, W.E. 1991. Cardiovascular risk factor levels in ethnic Hawaiians. *American Journal of Public Health* 81:164–167.

Gall, S.B., and Gall, T.L. (Eds.) 1993. Statistical Record of Asian Americans. Detroit: Gale Research Unit.

Gamble, V.N. 1994. Racial differentials in medical care: Implications for research on women. In: Women and Health Research: Ethical and Legal Issues of Including Women in Clinical Studies, Volume 2, A. Mastroianni, R. Faden, and D. Federman, eds. Washington, D.C.: National Academy Press.

Haenszel, W., and Kurihara, M. 1968. Studies of Japanese migrants, I. Mortality from cancer and other diseases among Japanese in the United States. *Journal of the National Cancer Institute* 40:43–68.

Hinds, M.W., Kolonel, L.N., Lee, J., and Hirohata, T. 1980. Associations between cancer incidence and alcohol/cigarette consumption among five ethnic groups in Hawaii. *British Journal of Cancer* 41:929–940.

Hurh, W.M., and Kim, K.C. 1982. Methodological problems in the study of Korean immigrants: Conceptual, interactional, sampling and interviewer training difficulties. Pp. 81–93 in: Methodological Problems in Minority Research, Occasional Paper No. 7, W.T. Liu, ed. Chicago: Pacific/Asian American Mental Health Research Center.

Kagan, A., Harris, B.R., Winkelstein, W., Johnson, K.G., Kato, H., Syme, S.L., Rhoads, G.G., Gay, M.L., Nichaman, M.Z., Hamilton, H.B., and Tillotson, J. 1974. Epidemiologic studies of coronary heart disease and stroke in Japanese men living in Japan, Hawaii and California: Demographic, physical, dietary and biochemical characteristics. *Journal of Chronic Disease* 27:345–364.

Kato, H., Tillotson, J., Nichaman, M.Z., Rhoads, G.G., and Hamilton, H.B. 1973. Epidemiologic studies of coronary heart disease and stroke in Japanese men living in Japan, Hawaii, and California: Serum lipids and diet. *American Journal of Epidemiology* 97:372–385.

King, H. 1975. Selected epidemiologic aspects of major disease and causes of death among Chinese in the United States and Asia. Pp. 487–550 in A. Kleinman, P.

Kunstadter, E.R. Alexander, and J.L. Gale, eds. Medicine in Chinese Cultures: Comparative Analysis of Health Care in Chinese and Other Societies. Pub. No. (NHI) 75-653. Washington, D.C.: Government Printing Office.

Klatsky, A.L., and Armstrong, M.A. 1991. Cardiovascular risk factors among Asian Americans living in Northern California. *American Journal of Public Health* 81:1423–1427.

Kleinman, J.C. 1990. Infant mortality among racial/ethnic minority groups, 1983–1984. *Mortality and Morbidity Weekly Report* 39(SS-3):31–39.

Kolonel, L.N., Hankin, J.H., Lee, J., Chu, S.Y., Nomura, A.M.Y., and Hinds, M.W. 1981. Nutrient intakes in relation to cancer incidence in Hawaii. *British Journal of Cancer* 44:332–339.

Li, D.K., Ni, H., Schwartz, S.M., and Daling, J.R. 1990. Secular change in birthweight among Southeast Asian immigrants to the United States. *American Journal of Public Health* 80:685–688.

Liu, W.T., and Yu, E.S.H. 1985. Asian/Pacific American elderly: Mortality differentials, Health status, and use of health Services. *Journal of Applied Gerontology* 4:35–64.

Lynberg, M., and Muin, J.K. 1990. Contribution of birth defects to infant mortality among racial/ethnic groups, United States, 1983. *Mortality and Morbidity Weekly Reports* 39(SS-3):1–11.

Reed, D., and Yano, K. 1987. Epidemiological studies of hypertension among elderly Japanese and Japanese Americans. *Asia-Pacific Journal of Public Health* 1:49–56.

Rhoads, G.G., and Feinleib, M. 1983. Serum triglyceride and risk of coronary heart disease, stroke, and total mortality in Japanese-American men. *Arteriosclerosis* 3:316–322.

Robertson, T.L., Kato, H., Rhoads, G.G., Kagan, A., Marmot, M., Syme, S.L., Gordon, T., Worth, R.M., Belsky, J.L., Dock, D.S., Miyanish, M., and Kawamoto, S. 1977. Epidemiologic studies of coronary heart disease and stroke in Japanese men living in Japan, Hawaii, and California. *American Journal of Cardiology* 39:239–243.

Stavig, G.R., Igra, A., and Leonard, A.R. 1984. Hypertension among Asians and Pacific Islanders in California. *American Journal of Epidemiology* 119:677–691.

Stemmermann, G.N., Chyou, P.H., Kagan, A., Nomura, A.M.Y., and Yano, K. 1991. Serum cholesterol and mortality among Japanese-American men. *Archives of Internal Medicine* 151:969–972.

Takeya, Y., Popper, J.S., Shimizu, Y., Kato, H., Rhoads, G.G., and Kagan, A. 1984. Epidemiologic studies of coronary heart disease and stroke in Japanese men living in Japan, Hawaii, and California: Incidence of stroke in Japan and Hawaii. *Stroke* 15:15–23.

Tillotson, J.L., Kato, H., Nichaman, M.Z., Miller, D.C., Gay, M.L., Johnson, K.G., and Rhoads, G.G. 1973. Epidemiology of coronary heart disease and stroke in Japanese men living in Japan, Hawaii, and California: methodology for comparison of diet. *The American Journal of Clinical Nutrition* 26:177–184.

U.S. Department of Health and Human Services. 1991. Protection of Human Subjects, OPPR Report: Title 45 C.F.R. Part 46, Rev. June 18. Pp. 1–17.

U.S. Department of Health and Human Services. 1990. Healthy People 2000, DHHS Pub. No. (PHS) 91-50213.

U.S. Department of Health and Human Services. 1979. The Belmont Report: Ethical

Principles and Guidelines for the Protection of Human Subjects of Research. Pp. 1–8.

Wolfensberger, W. 1967. Ethical issues in research with human subjects. *Science* 155(3758):47–61.

Yano, K., Reed, D.M., Curb, J.D., Hankin, H.H., and Albers, J.J. 1986. Biological and dietary correlates of plasma lipids and lipoproteins among elderly Japanese men in Hawaii. *Arteriosclerosis* 6(4):422–433.

Yano, K., and MacLean, C.J. 1989. The incidence and prognosis of unrecognized myocardial infarction in the Honolulu, Hawaii, Heart Program. *Archives of Internal Medicine* 149:1528–1532.

Yu, E.S.H., and Liu, W.T. 1992. U.S. National Health Data on Asian Americans and Pacific Islanders: A Research Agenda for the 1990s. *American Journal of Public Health* 82,12:1645–1652.

Yu, E.S.H., and Liu, W.T. 1986. Methodological problems and policy implications in Vietnamese refugee research. *International Migration Review* 20(2):483–501.

Yu, E.S.H. 1986. Health of the Chinese elderly in America. *Research on Aging* 8:84–109.

Inclusion of Latino Women in Clinical and Research Studies: Scientific Suggestions for Assuring Legal and Ethical Integrity

Ruth E. Zambrana

In research, legal and ethical issues are embedded in the scientific process, that is, in the current paradigms and methodological approaches used in the study of racial and ethnic groups in the United States. The purpose of this commentary is to discuss the methodological and conceptual areas relevant to the inclusion of Latino women in research and clinical studies. The main issues in this area have been the limited recognition of the importance of the use of racial and ethnic identifiers in investigations, narrow conceptual paradigms, and inappropriate data collection procedures.

The lack of adequate descriptions of the respondents in a study (the study sample) has violated the principles of scientific method. There is a current debate regarding how to measure racial and ethnic identifiers, what their importance and meaning is, and the potential negative implications in standardizing race and ethnic identifiers (King and Williams, 1993). There is clear evidence that race and ethnic identifiers are merely one set of indicators that are highly interrelated with socioeconomic indicators (which most investigators also are generally reluctant to carefully measure). There is a consensus in the health services research field that poverty or low-income status is the strongest predictor of the use of health services and health outcome. Yet there is limited understanding of the complex processes and factors which influence the pathways to unfavorable health outcome in Latino groups. In addition, socioeconomic status and race and ethnicity must be adequately measured as separate and independent variables to examine their effects on health behaviors, psychosocial factors, and institutional factors (access, cost, and quality of services) (Williams, 1990).

The 1990 PHS/NIH policy ruling that required the inclusion of racial and ethnic groups and women forced the scientific community to examine issues of inclusion of these groups in studies, but did not provide guidelines for determining adequate sample size of these groups in a study. Thus there remains the central concern that current and future studies may not include sufficient numbers of Hispanic women for subgroup differences to be estimated, a methodological flaw rendering study data scientifically and practically unusable.

LATINO HEALTH: A BRIEF OVERVIEW

There has been an unprecedented increase in Latino and immigrant populations in the United States since 1970. In 1990, the number of Latinos in the United States reached 22 million (9.2 percent of the total population). It is expected that Latinos will continue to grow at the rate of 33 percent over the next decade. The Latino population is quite diverse, the largest group being Mexican Americans (63 percent), who are concentrated mainly in Texas, New Mexico, Arizona, and California; Puerto Ricans (15 percent), in New York, Boston, Chicago, and Washington, D.C.; Central and South American and other Hispanics (18 percent); and Cubans (6 percent), concentrated in Florida.

Immigration to the United States has been greatest among Mexican and Central American refugees owing to political and economic events in their country of origin. The Immigration and Naturalization Service (INS) recorded 2.7 million Latin American immigrants to the United States between 1960 and 1970 (Puerto Ricans, who are U.S. citizens, are not included in this count), with an increase of about 500,000 per year. At present one-third of all births in California are to foreign-born Hispanic women.

In 1990, the poverty rate for Hispanic persons was 28.1 percent and these rates were higher for families with a female head (48.3 percent). Current knowledge in the area of Latino health suggests that the health of Latino women, children, and their families seriously affects and is affected by their socioeconomic position in society. The following points provide a brief profile of Latinos in the United States and depicts subgroup differences.

1. The majority of Latino families tend to be larger than non-Hispanic white families (4.4 compared to 1.8), less educated ($M = 8.8$ years of schooling for Mexican immigrants, 11.9 for those of native Mexican origin, and 13.2 for Anglos), at a lower income level ($21,800 vs. $42,000 for non-Hispanic whites), younger (mean age 23 years vs. 31 years for non-Hispanic whites) and less likely to have medical insurance. It is estimated that 53 percent of Latinos have no health insurance in California, partly as a result of the types of work they do

as farm workers, domestic workers, and day workers.

2. Latino women have higher fertility, tend to begin childbearing at younger ages, and are three times more likely than non-Hispanic white or African American women to delay prenatal care, that is, initiate care in the third trimester. However, among all poor and racial and ethnic women only about 58 percent initiate care in the first trimester, compared to 80 percent of the general population.

3. Delayed use of health care, organizational and financial barriers, knowledge, attitudes, and beliefs have all been documented as a set of interrelated factors that seriously influence the health outcomes of Latino groups. These barriers are heightened by immigrant status.

4. The leading causes of death in Latino women are diseases of the heart, diabetes, and cancer (breast, lung). For example, females of Mexican origin account for 48 percent of all deaths from cancer in Texas. However, the prevalence and incidence of these diseases varies significantly across Latino subgroups (USDHHS, 1985; Frank-Stromberg, 1991; Desenclos and Hahn, 1992).

Existing Data Sets

At present there are few data sets that include sufficient number by Latino subgroups to conduct any meaningful analyses (USPHS, 1992; Amaro, 1993). In 1990, extensive data were published from the Hispanic Health and Nutrition Examination Survey (H-HANES), undertaken by the National Center for Health Statistics (see *JAMA,* 1991; *AJPH,* 1991). H-HANES is the first large-scale health survey to target the Latino population in the United States, specifically Mexican Americans, mainland Puerto Ricans, and Cuban Americans. The total sample comprised 12,000 Latinos from the three ethnic subgroups, who lived in three geographic areas (namely, five southwestern states, New York City and its surrounding area, and Dade County, Florida). Although the value of the data obtained by H-HANES should not be underestimated, it is still crucial to note that these data were collected during 1982–1984. Thus, although this database is one of the largest comprehensive studies regarding the health status of Latinos, it has taken almost ten years for these data to become available.

In spite of the documented differences found in disease patterns among Latino subgroups, current plans for the H-HANES will include only Mexican Americans. In its most recent report, the PHS documented that most record-based surveys have no entry for "race and ethnicity," which severely limits the availability of tabulations about racial and ethnic populations in the United States (USPHS, 1992:17). With specific reference to Hispanics, vital statistics data are even more limited. Although there was a revision to the U.S. Standard Birth and Death Certificate in 1989 with clear race and specific ethnic identifiers, there is no standard format established for the states to report these data (USPHS, 1992:27).

Heterogeneity within the Hispanic population clearly requires that data be collected by subgroup and analyzed separately. Data from the H-HANES and national birth data show distinct differences in patterns of clinical outcome by subgroup, that is, Puerto Ricans, Mexican Americans and Cuban Americans (*JAMA,* 1991). In addition, there are distinct differences between Mexican immigrants and Mexican Americans. These differences are related to place of birth (nativity), socioeconomic status, geographic context, and lifestyle behaviors. These variables must be incorporated and measured in future research studies.

LIMITATIONS OF EXISTING RESEARCH APPROACHES

The scientific approach to understanding the complex needs of Latino women, particularly in the field of health, has been driven by a rigid, narrow, and homogeneous set of principles which have not permitted the exploration of diversity in the health trajectories of these women. The fields of health services research, biomedical research, demography, and social epidemiology have narrowly and inconsistently defined the parameters of disease patterns as unidimensional, that is, occurring outside the context of a social environment, a psychosocial context, and a family context (Williams, 1990; Lillie-Blanton et al., 1993). The developmental life of a disease, the effectiveness of interventions and procedures used, and the patient's clinical outcome must be measured within the social, cultural, and psychological context of the individual's life. Thus the recognition that biologic, psychological, social, and cultural factors interact with clinical processes needs to inform the paradigm that seeks to understand the particular disease patterns, the effectiveness of interventions, and the course of illness in Latino groups.

Past and current research endeavors have exhibited several features: (1) they are generally individualistic, that is, guided by a principal investigator; (2) there is a limited value of the role of collaboration, either across disciplines or with the community or subjects; and (3) the experiences of many researchers are not practice- or community-based. Thus there is a need to improve our conceptual paradigms, methodological approaches, and data collection procedures (Zambrana, 1992).

There have been few guidelines and operational definitions to guide the investigations on low-income Latino groups (Zambrana, 1991, 1992). This has seriously impeded comparability across studies and across national data sets (USPHS, 1992). Research on Latinos, and women of this group, need to incorporate the following characteristics:

1. A sensitivity to and a real world knowledge of the problems experienced by the specific Latino group under study. For example, the socioenvironmental context and the availability and quality of health services varies by geographic region, socioeconomic status, rural/urban setting and immigration status among different subgroups of Latinos.

2. Adequate measurement of study variables, using a set of cross-culturally and socioeconomically appropriate instruments that have been pretested through a set of scientific and systematic steps to assure reliability and validity of the data.

3. Use of an analytic model that permits the examination of the direct effects of race, ethnicity, socioeconomic status, and nativity on health behaviors, psychosocial factors, and their interactions with institutional variables and their relationship to clinical outcomes of interest.

4. Measurement of the role of cultural beliefs with reference to health-seeking behaviors and the specific clinical conditions.

Thus a more comprehensive biopsychosocial model must inform and guide future studies which seek to better understand the intricate relationships among these variables and their influence on the health status of Latino women. Data collection procedures are integral to assuring reliable and valid data. Thus, in the design of a study focusing on Latino women, the investigators must understand that context and work closely with appropriate informants of that community so that they can develop appropriate and cross-culturally and linguistically sensitive instruments to collect data, develop appropriate procedures to involve the community, identify representative groups of women in conjunction with community experts, and involve community providers and experts as well as potential subjects in the development and conduct of the study (McGraw et al., 1992).

HUMAN PROTECTION PROCEDURES AND INFORMED CONSENT

Efforts to develop mechanisms to protect the rights of research subjects have improved dramatically in the last two decades. The underlying principles guiding the legislative mandate were that potential research subjects be informed of the nature of the study and its potential risks and benefits to themselves and their community, and that they willingly and in full understanding of the research objectives participate and cooperate with the research protocol. The key elements of the informed consent process include disclosure of information, understanding of information, and decision making (Gray and Osterweis, 1986:548). These procedures did not provide any additional guidelines to investigators when dealing with racial and ethnic groups who had a history of being uninformed experimental subjects in the past, or when conducting studies with language and cultural minorities and individuals with limited education. Thus there are three central areas that require attention in human subject protection procedures for Latino women: prior history as research subjects, language, and education with respect to appropriateness of measurement and instruments, and representation on institutional review boards to assure that ethical procedures are instituted.

In the study of Latino women, there is an extensive history of reproductive abuse. For example, Puerto Rican women were used as experimental subjects in early clinical trials of birth control pills, intrauterine devices, and Emko contraceptive cream in the 1950s. The long-range consequence of these experiments has been high rates of cervical cancer among Puerto Rican women. Furthermore, there is documented evidence of high rates of sterilization of Puerto Rican women, both in New York and Puerto Rico, and Mexican-American women in California and the Southwest (Lopez, 1987; Vasquez, 1988). These and other documented failures by the scientific community (Gamble, 1993) to protect the rights of poor and Latino women have contributed to a lack of trust of many in the Latino community and to a resistance to providing access for investigations.

However, equally important has been the lack of sensitivity of many investigators to issues of Spanish translation and literacy in the translation of instruments and informed consent procedures. A careful review of the Spanish translations of instruments and informed consent procedures immediately reveals several problems: almost all are direct translations of the English, which are generally neither culturally nor linguistically appropriate to low-income Latino groups. The language is often too sophisticated, and thus educationally and linguistically inappropriate. In terms of school completion, only about 60 percent of Latinos graduate from high school in the United States and many immigrants, especially from Mexico and Central America, have limited education.

The method most often used in translating instruments into Spanish is a back or direct language translation technique which makes a number of assumptions that may threaten the validity of the data: (a) the cultural meaning of the words exists in both cultures; (b) the grammatical structure of the language is the same; (c) the existing instruments are adequate for use among low-income and culturally or racially distinct populations; (d) anyone who knows "Spanish" can translate since Spanish is the mother tongue of all. This last assumption is the most damaging since it ignores different meanings of Spanish words in different subgroups, educational differences, and colloquialisms by region and group.

In effect, Spanish translation should be reviewed by individuals who are from the ethnic group under study and who have firsthand knowledge and experience of the target population. Methodologically, two approaches can be used: a panel of bilingual individuals of the particular Latino subgroup under study, who have experience in working with the community, can participate in the review and translation of the instrument to assure correct colloquial words, symbolic meaning, word structure; and pretests of the instruments with subjects who have comparable characteristics to study population must be conducted. These approaches can replace or supplement back translation methodologies (Zambrana, 1992).

Institutional review boards (IRBs) at existing research institutions must judge the acceptability of the research protocol regarding risk, informed consent, confidentiality, and mechanisms to assure that the protocol is understood by the subjects and that subjects freely consent without coercion or perceived threat. In a study conducted by the National Commission for the Protection of Human Subjects in the late 1970s, it was found that IRBs did not appear effective in carefully monitoring forms for inclusion of important information. Forms "tended to be unrealistically difficult to read, and there was "great institutional variation in operation of IRBs." Although in 1983, the President's Commission "recommended that more active educational programs be instituted by the federal government" (p. 548), the central point made by these authors is that IRBs are an example of "the capture of the regulatory process by the regulated" (p. 549).

Thus members of existing IRBs at research institutions are highly unlikely to have representatives who are familiar with particular Latino groups, with cultural and language issues related to these groups, or with appropriate research paradigms or cross-cultural instrumentation and measurement issues. Thus there may be significant barriers to the assurances of the inclusion of significant number of Latino women and most importantly to the development of ethically sound procedures for their inclusion.

Although there has been a clear recognition of the increased racial and ethnic diversity in our society, the scientific community continues to be entrenched in a scientific method that measures homogeneity and ignores the particular life context of communities in which individuals outside the middle class and dominant culture conduct their lives. There is a pressing need to shift our paradigms in the study of Latino women and to conduct research in ways that assure the ethical integrity of the subjects and the scientific findings (see King and Williams, 1993).

RECOMMENDATIONS

The following five recommendations are integrally related to assuring the ethical integrity and scientific validity of data when including Latino women in research studies:

1. Develop a more comprehensive biopsychosocial model which examines the influence of socioeconomic status, ethnicity, race, nativity (place of birth),

and cultural attitudes and beliefs on access to health services, compliance, and clinical outcome. A model can begin to guide systematic research in the area of Latino health, especially Latino women's health. Conceptual models are the cornerstone of a set of empirically valid research questions and an appropriate design and sampling procedures.

2. Design studies with adequate sample size of Latino women in relevant research studies to assure the analytic ability to examine data by age and ethnic subgroup, to conduct planned comparisons across Latino subgroups, and to establish baseline data for future investigations.

3. Develop mechanisms to foster a significant number of Latino investigators (who are familiar with the local cultural and geographic community) in this effort who will serve as principal investigators and members on IRBs to assure cultural, linguistic, and educational sensitivity in methodological procedures and instrument development.

4. Develop clear and required guidelines for the inclusion of the appropriate groups in the community to help identify appropriate Latino women for study, to involve the women in designing the study, such as in focus groups, and to better understand the study within the community context and in the pre- and pilot-testing of the instruments as subjects and as interviewers.

5. Assemble interdisciplinary teams so that both qualitative and quantitative methodological approaches can be appropriately used to insure contextual understanding of the community, cross-culturally sensitive instrument development, and scientifically useful data both in terms of scientific knowledge building and policy and program relevance to the community under study.

Presently the Latino population in the United States is growing at unprecedented rates and there is a compelling need to generate data that are usable in the community to develop programs and policies that can appropriately address the emerging health issues and problems of Latino women.

To this end, data must be generated which adequately captures their health status and those factors that differentially influence their clinical outcomes.

REFERENCES

Amaro, Hortensia. 1993. Using National Health Data Systems To Inform Hispanic Women's Health. Paper presented at the National Center for Health Statistics Public Health Conference on Records and Statistics. Washington, D.C. July 19–21.

American Medical Association. 1991. *JAMA,* Hispanic Health Issue 265(2):161–296.

Desenclos, J. A. and Hahn, R.A. 1992. Years of Potential Life Lost Before Age 65, by Race, Hispanic Origin, and Sex—United States, 1986–1988. *MMWR,* 42 (November).

Frank-Stromborg, M. 1991. Changing Demographics in the United States. *Cancer* 67:1772– 778.

Gamble, V.N., and Blustein, B.E. 1994. Racial Differentials in Medical Care: Implications for Research on Women. In A.C. Mastroianni, R. Faden, and R.D. Federman, eds. *Women and Health Research: Ethical and Legal Issues of Including Women in Clinical Studies, Vol. 2.* Washington, D.C.: National Academy Press.

Gray, B.H., and Osterweis, M. 1986. Ethical Issues in a Social Context. In Linda Aiken and David Mechanic, eds. *Application of Social Science to Clinical Medicine and Health Policy.* New Brunswick, New Jersey: Rutgers University Press.

King, G., and Williams, D.R. 1993. Race and Health: A Multidimensional Approach to African American Health. Department of Community Medicine and Health Care, School of Medicine, University of Connecticut Health Center. Farmington, CT. (unpublished manuscript)

Lillie, M., Martinez, R.M., Taylor, A.K., and Robinson, B.G. 1993. Latino and African American Women: Continuing Disparities in Health. *International Journal of Health Services,* 23(3):555–584.

Lopez, I.O. 1987. Sterilization among Puerto Rican Women in New York City: Public Policy and Social Constraints. In Leith Mullings (ed.), *Cities of the United States: Studies in Urban Anthropology.* New York: Columbia University Press.

McGraw, S.A., McKinlay, J.B., Crawford, S.A., Costa, L.A., and Cohen, D.L. 1992. Health Survey Methods with Minority Populations: Some Lessons from Recent Experience. *Ethnicity and Disease,* 2:273–287.

National Commission for the Protection of Human Subjects of Biomedical and Behavioral Research, 1978. Report and Recommendations Institutional Review Boards. Washington, D.C.: U.S. Government Printing Office.

Trevion, F.M., Falcon, A. P., and C.A. Stroup-Benham (eds.) 1990. Hispanic Health and Nutrition Examination Survey, 1982–84: Findings on Health Status and Health Care Needs. American Journal of Public Health 80: Supplement.

U.S. Department of Health and Human Services. 1986. Report of the Secretary's Task Force on Black and Minority Health. *Infant Mortality and Low Birth Weight,* 6.

U.S. Department of Health and Human Services. 1985. Report of the Public Health Service Task Force on Women's Health Issues. *Women's Health,* 2.

U.S. Public Health Service. 1992. Improving Minority Health Statistics. Report of the Public Health Service Task Force on Minority Health.

Vasquez-Calzada, J.L. 1988. La Populacion de Puerto Rico y su Trajectoria Historica. San Juan: Escuela Graduada de Salud Publica, Recinto de Ciencias Medicas, Universidad de Puerto Rico.

Williams, D.R. 1990. Socioeconomic Differentials in Health. *Social Psychology Quarterly,* 53(2):81–99.

Zambrana, R.E. 1992. The relationship between use of health care services and health status: dilemmas in measuring medical outcome in low-income and racial ethnic populations. In M.L. Grady and H.A. Schwartz (eds.), *Medical Effectiveness Research Data Methods.* Rockville, MD: U.S. Department of Health and Human Services. Pp. 103-114.

Zambrana, R.E. 1991. Cross-cultural methodological strategies in the study of low-income racial ethnic populations. In M.L. Grady (ed.), *AHCPR Conference Proceedings—Primary Care Research: Theory and Methods.* Rockville, MD: U.S. Department of Health and Human Services. Pp. 221-227.

Appendix

Author Biographies

Leslie Z. Benet, Ph.D., is Professor and Chairman in the Department of Pharmacy at the University of California, San Francisco. He earned his Ph.D. from the University of California, and in 1987 was awarded a Pharm. D. *honoris causa* from Uppsala University in Sweden. His current research interests and more than 270 publications are in the areas of pharmacokinetics, drug metabolism, and pharmacodynamics of immunosuppressive agents, organic nitrates, and NSAIDs. In 1987, Dr. Benet was elected to membership in the Institute of Medicine of the National Academy of Sciences. He currently serves the IOM as Chair of the Committee on Antiprogestins: Assessing the Science, and as a member of the Forum on Drug Development and Regulation.

Chloe E. Bird, Ph.D., is a Postdoctoral Fellow in the Joint Program in Society and Health at the New England Medical Center and Harvard School of Public Health. She earned her Ph.D. in Sociology from the University of Illinois at Urbana-Champaign. She has published on gender stratification in the labor force and the social determinants of gender differences in health. Her current research interests include women's representation in the health professions, the effects of the division of household labor and perceived fairness of role allocation on men's and women's mental health, and the social and economic consequences of parenthood for men's and women's health.

Bonnie Ellen Blustein, Ph.D., completed her undergraduate work in philosophy at Radcliffe College (Harvard University) and earned her Ph.D. in History and Sociology of Science at the University of Pennsylvania. She has taught U.S. history, the history of science, and the history of medicine at the University of

241

Wisconsin-Madison, Northwestern University, the University of Louisville, and elsewhere. Dr. Blustein is the author of *Preserve Your Love for Science: Life of William A. Hammond, American Neurologist* (1991) and *Educating for Health and Prevention: A History of the Department of Community and Preventive Medicine at the (Woman's) Medical College of Pennsylvania* (1993). She has also published numerous articles. Dr. Blustein is presently completing a book on the history of neurology in America, 1863-1945. Her other current research interests include intersections of race/class, and ways in which neurology and neuroscience have been invoked in discussions of social policy issues.

Sandra D. Cassard, Sc.D., earned her Sc.D. in Health Policy and Management from the Johns Hopkins University School of Hygiene and Public Health. Her research interests are in the areas of women's health and the relationship between health care services and patient outcomes.

R. Alta Charo, J.D., is Assistant Professor of Law and Medical Ethics at the University of Wisconsin Schools of Law and Medicine. She holds honors degrees in biology (Harvard-Radcliffe) and law (Columbia), and has served as Associate Director of the Legislative Drafting Research Fund, Legal Analyst for the Biological Applications Program of the Congressional Office of Technology Assessment, and Policy Analyst for the Office of Population of the U.S. Agency for International Development. Professor Charo has served on the steering committee for the International Association for Bioethics and currently serves on the executive boards of the Alan Guttmacher Institute and International Projects Assistance Services. She is currently working on a series of articles concerning reproductive choice in light of enhanced genetic knowledge, and has begun a project on the role of biology as ideology in the political and legal arenas.

Ellen Wright Clayton, J.D., M.D., is a graduate of Yale Law School and Harvard Medical School. She is currently Assistant Professor of Pediatrics and Assistant Professor of Law at Vanderbilt University, as well as a Charles E. Culpepper Foundation Scholar in Medical Humanities. Her research interests include informed consent, the doctor-patient relationship, and factors that lead patients to sue their physicians. She also has a longstanding interest in the impact of new reproductive technologies on women and in the legal, ethical, and social implications of technologies that make it possible to diagnose and treat genetic disorders.

Debra A. DeBruin, Ph.D., is Assistant Professor of Philosophy at the University of Illinois at Chicago. She earned her Ph.D. at the University of Pittsburgh. Her primary research interests lie in the areas of ethics, social and political philosophy, and the philosophy of feminism.

Elizabeth Fee, Ph.D., is Professor of History and Health Policy at the Johns Hopkins School of Hygiene and Public Health, and holds a joint appointment in the Johns Hopkins Institute for the History of Medicine. She is the author of *Disease and Discovery* (Johns Hopkins University Press, 1987), editor of *Women and Health* (Baywood, 1983), and co-editor, with Roy M. Acheson, of *A History of Education in Public Health* (Oxford University Press, 1991). She is also co-editor, with Daniel M. Fox, of *AIDS: The Burdens of History* (University of California Press, 1992), and serves as contributing editor for history for the *American Journal of Public Health*. She teaches courses at Johns Hopkins on the History of Public Health, the History of Health Policy, and Women's Health.

Ellen Flannery, J.D., is Partner in the law firm of Covington and Burling in Washington, D.C. Her practice includes pharmaceutical and medical device law. She has been a Lecturer in Food and Drug Law at the University of Virginia Law School from 1984-1990, and has written several articles on the regulation of drugs and medical devices. Ms. Flannery is Chair of the American Bar Association (ABA) Section on Science and Technology and Vice Chair of the Food and Drug Law Committee of the ABA's Business Law Section. Ms. Flannery earned her J.D. cum laude from Boston University School of Law, where she served as Editor-in-Chief of the Law Review, and an A.B. cum Laude from Mount Holyoke College.

Vanessa Northington Gamble, M.D., Ph.D., is an associate Professor in the Departments of History of Medicine, Preventive Medicine, and Family Medicine at the University of Wisconsin. She teaches courses on health policy, race and American medicine, and the history of American medicine. She obtained a M.D. and a Ph.D. in the History and Sociology of Science from the University of Pennsylvania. Her primary area of research is the history of race and racism in American medicine. She has written and lectured extensively on the topic. Her book *Making A Place For Ourselves: The Black Hospital Movement, 1920-1945,* will be published next year by Oxford University Press. She is presently working on a history of black women physicians and a study of how issues of race have influenced American medical thought.

Sanford N. Greenberg, J.D., is an associate in the law firm of Covington & Burling in Washington, D.C. He specializes in environmental insurance coverage and federal and state health care funding. Mr. Greenberg received his J.D. with highest honors from the George Washington University National Law Center, where he was Editor-in-Chief of the Law Review. He received his A.B. from Princeton University, where he was elected to Phi Beta Kappa. Mr. Greenberg also has earned an M.A. and Ph.D. in Political Science from the University of California at Berkeley under fellowships from the Danforth Foundation and

National Science Foundation. Prior to associating with Covington & Burling in 1991, Mr. Greenberg was a law clerk on the U.S. Court of Appeals for the Seventh Circuit.

Tracy Johnson, M.A., is Project Manager for the Society for the Advancement of Women's Health Research at the Bass & Howes consulting firm. She holds an M.A. in Religious and Biomedical Ethics. Her research and publications have focused on women's health and have included such topics as women in clinical trials, sexual assault, RU486, cocaine use in pregnancy, prenatal diagnosis, and women in academic medicine. Ms. Johnson has also served as the Community Education Coordinator for the Sexual Assault Resource Agency in Charlottesville, Virginia, and as Project Manager at Commonwealth Clinical Systems, a data processing company for Medicare Peer Review Organizations (PROs).

Robert J. Levine, M.D., is Professor of Medicine (medical ethics) and Lecturer in Pharmacology at Yale University School of Medicine. He is Chairperson of the Institutional Review Board at Yale-New Haven Medical Center and a Fellow of the Hastings Center and of the American College of Physicians. Dr. Levine is Editor of *IRB: A Review of Human Subjects Research* and has served as a consultant to several federal and international agencies involved in the development of policy for the protection of human subjects. He is author of numerous publications including *Ethics and Regulation of Research* (2nd ed., 1986).

Barbara W. Lex, Ph.D., M.P.H., is Associate Professor of Psychiatry/ Anthropology in the Alcohol and Drug Abuse Research Center of the Department of Psychiatry of Harvard Medical School. She received her Ph.D. in (medical) anthropology from Syracuse University in 1969, and began work in alcohol and drug abuse problems. Dr. Lex received her M.P.H. from the Harvard School of Public Health in 1982, having focused her studies on psychiatric epidemiology, health care promotion, and public health policy and management. Throughout her career Dr. Lex has published and reviewed several publications on the epidemiology of alcohol effects on women, youth, elderly, and minority group members (American Indians, Hispanics, and African Americans).

Wendy K. Mariner, J.D., LL.M., M.P.H., is Professor of Health Law at Boston University Schools of Medicine and Public Health. She earned her J.D. from Columbia University, her LL.M. in Taxation from New York University, and her M.P.H. from Harvard School of Public Health. Before joining Boston University, Professor Mariner taught Health Law at Harvard School of Public Health and Harvard Medical School, where she remains a Lecturer in Social

Medicine. At Boston University, she is a senior faculty member in the Law, Medicine, and Ethics Program and faculty advisor for the J.D.-M.P.H. joint degree program. Professor Mariner has been named an American Foundation for AIDS Research/Michael Bennett Scholar to study AIDS and the future of legal entitlement to health care.

Vanessa Merton, J.D., is Associate Dean for Clinical Education and Professor of Law at Pace University School of Law. Formerly a professor and Director of Clinical Programs at City University of New York Law School and New York University Law School, she currently teaches health law courses and supervises the Health Law Clinic. Professor Merton was the founding chairperson of the Institutional Review Board of the Community Research Initiative of New York, one of the first centers for community-based biomedical research on AIDS, and the first Associate for Law at the Hastings Center Institute for Society, Ethics, and the Life Sciences. She has lectured and written extensively on issues of biomedical and professional ethics, health law, and professional education.

Janet L. Mitchell, M.D., M.P.H., is Chief of Perinatology at Harlem Hospital Center and Assistant Professor at Columbia University School of Public Health and College of Physicians and Surgeons. She earned her M.D. from the Howard University School of Medicine and her M.P.H. from the Harvard University School of Public Health. Dr. Mitchell directs the largest prenatal program for substance abusing pregnant women in New York City. Her career interests include substance abuse by pregnant women, women and AIDS, adolescent pregnancy, and infant mortality.

Jonathan D. Moreno, Ph.D., is Professor of Pediatrics and of Medicine (Bioethics) and Director of the Division of Humanities in Medicine at the SUNY Health Sciences Center in Brooklyn. He is also an Adjunct Associate of the Hastings Center. Currently, Dr. Moreno is collaborating on a clinical ethics textbook and writing a book on consensus in bioethics.

Janice Racine Norris, M.A., graduated from Smith College in 1984 with an A.B. in European History. She received a M.A. in European Medieval History from Boston College in 1987, and is currently a doctoral candidate at Binghamton University where her dissertation topic focused on Anglo-Saxon women of the late sixth to mid-ninth centuries and their participation in the Christianization of England. Ms. Norris has a long-standing interest in contemporary women's issues, and in recent years has developed an interest in Native Americans of the Southwest.

John Robertson, J.D., is Thomas Watt Gregory Professor of Law at the University of Texas School of Law at Austin. A graduate of Dartmouth College and Harvard Law School, he has written widely on law and bioethics issues, including the book, *The Rights of the Critically Ill* and numerous articles on reproductive rights, organ transplantation, and human experimentation. A Fellow of the Hastings Center, he has served on a federal Task Force on Organ Transplantation, on the National Institutes of Health Panel on Fetal Tissues Transplantation Research, and on the Ethics Committee of the American Fertility Society. His new book, *Autonomy and Ambivalence: Reproductive Technology and the Limits of Procreative Liberty*, will be published in 1994 by Princeton University Press.

Susan Sherwin, Ph.D., is Professor of Philosophy and Women's Studies at Dalhousie University, Halifax, Nova Scotia. She earned a Ph.D. in Philosophy from Stanford University, and was a Postdoctoral Fellow in the Moral Problems in Medicine Project, Case Western Reserve University. Ms. Sherwin is the author of *No Longer Patient: Feminist Ethics and Health Care* (Temple University Press, 1992).

Bonnie Steinbock, Ph.D., is Associate Professor and Chair of the Department of Philosophy at the State University of New York at Albany. Her publications are in applied ethics, primarily bioethics. She is the author of *Life Before Birth: The Moral and Legal Status of Embryos and Fetuses* (Oxford University Press, 1992).

Diane Stoy, R.N., Ed.D., is Operations Director of the Lipid Research Clinic at the George Washington University, where she is also Adjunct Assistant Professor in the Department of Health Care Sciences. Ms. Stoy has designed and directed recruitment and adherence programs for a variety of collaborative clinical studies involving women, such as studies with young women and oral contraceptives, postmenopausal women and hormone replacement, and elderly women and cholesterol-lowering medications.

Carol S. Weisman, Ph.D., is Professor of Health Policy and Management at the Johns Hopkins School of Hygiene and Public Health. She holds a Ph.D. in Social Relations from Johns Hopkins. She has conducted research on a variety of issues related to women's health, including studies of women's use of contraception and cancer screening services; provision of fertility-control services to women; gender differences in physician-patient communication; and effects of shift work on women's health. She is currently studying prevention of unintended pregnancy and STDs among adolescent and young adult men and women in Baltimore.

Elena S. H. Yu, Ph.D., M.P.H., is Professor of Public Health in the Division of Epidemiology and Biostatistics of the Graduate School of Public Health at San Diego State University. Dr. Yu has conducted research in Mainland China, Hong Kong, and the United States in the areas of minority and women's health, aging and dementia, and caregiving and caregiver's burden. She has published numerous scientific articles in the areas of epidemiology and neurology. In 1984 and 1985, Dr. Yu served as a consultant to the Secretary of Health and Human Services' Task Force on Black and Minority Health. In 1993, she served as a consultant to the Centers for Disease Control on the issue of measurements and uses of race and ethnicity in public health.

Ruth E. Zambrana, Ph.D.,, is Associate Professor of Social Welfare at UCLA (on leave). She is currently serving as a Senior Research Scientist at the Agency for Health Care Policy and Research, Center for Medical Effectiveness Research in Rockville, Maryland. Her research areas of interest are in racial and ethnic differences in factors which influence health status, family and children's health, and pregnancy outcome in low-income groups.